# Intermittent Diet for Women Over 50

*The Complete Guide for Intermittent Fasting Diet & Quick Weight Loss After 50, Easy Book for Senior Beginners, Including Week Diet Plan + Meal Ideas*

**Dr. Suzanne Ramos Hughes, Amy Ryan**

# Table of Contents

# Introduction

When a woman approaches a certain age, her body starts changing as the aging process kicks in. Women over fifty become high-risk targets for various health issues and start to find it harder to maintain their weight.

There has been scientific interest in intermittent fasting as research has started to uncover the numerous benefits of it. Post-menopause causes many changes in a woman including increased belly fat, depression, muscle pain, and joint pain. Women are moreover at more considerable risk for diabetes and cardiovascular disease. These are just a few of the symptoms that can be associated with a metabolic syndrome which is closely related to insulin resistance and prediabetes.

Research has shown that intermittent fasting in women over fifty could possibly reduce the risk of diabetes and may ease muscle and joint pain, especially lower back pain. It could, in addition, produce a positive anti-aging effect which is an added bonus along with better weight control to cut down on belly fat.

# Chapter 1: Introduction to the Intermittent Fasting Diet

Before you start any diet or drastically change your eating pattern, it is always advisable to seek the advice of a medical professional. This is especially true if you have an existing condition, as when there is fasting involved it may interfere with your medication or health.

**Benefits of Intermittent Fasting**

Heightens your insulin sensitivity

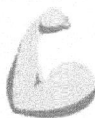

Increases growth hormone secretion for strong muscles

Lengthens your lifespan

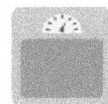

Helps with weight loss

## What is the Intermittent Fasting Diet?

Intermittent fasting (IF) is when a person refrains from eating during certain hours of the day. During the hours that the person is not fasting, they eat a healthy, regimented diet. The intermittent fasting diet is not so much of a diet but a lifestyle change.

Some of the more popular intermittent fasting methods are two to three days a week, alternate days, or daily during set hours. The thing about the intermittent fasting diet is that there is no need for counting calories, macronutrients, or cutting down on certain foods.

There are no set rules other than not eating certain set rules, and you can eat what you like during the time window in which you are not fasting. During the time when you are fasting, you can drink water, tea, and coffee.

Intermittent fasting is a diet that can be used to lose weight, enhance body composition, and decrease body fat. It has been known to have a lot of other health benefits, especially for women in middle age.

## History of Intermittent Fasting Diet

The father of modern medicine, Hippocrates of Cos, who lived between 460 BCE to 375 BCE, practiced fasting. Fasting an ancient method of healing along with apple cider vinegar. Plutarch was an ancient Greek historian and a writer, he also wrote about fasting rather than using medicine. Even Aristotle and his mentor Plato practiced and believed in fasting. (Fasting — A History Part 1, n.d.)

Fasting has been called the 'physician' within as all animals as well as humans tend to turn away from food when they are sick.

If you have ever been really sick you will know that the last thing you think of is food. It is as if fasting is ingrained into a person's DNA, a natural instinctive reaction to sickness as old as time.

After a large meal, the body reduces blood flow to the brain as it pushes more blood to the digestive system to help it digest a large meal. Fasting was thought to improve cognitive abilities by the ancient Greeks. But it was not only the ancient Greeks and great philosophers that believed in fasting but the founder of toxicology, Philip Paracelsus did too.

Fasting has been used for many other reasons besides medical or losing weight as well. It has also been used for spiritual purposes, religious purposes, purification, cleansing, and to make statements for a cause.

Fasting has been around for many years and will be around for many more years as scientists have now started to take an interest in its many benefits. Our ancient ancestors that were hunter-gatherers had to go out looking for food each day. Sometimes there was no food to be found and so they would go for long periods without eating. As a result, the human body evolved and adapted to be able to go without food for days at a time.

The body functions better when it has been deprived of food for a couple of hours as it gives it a chance to do some in-house cleaning.

# Chapter 2: Types of Intermittent Fasting

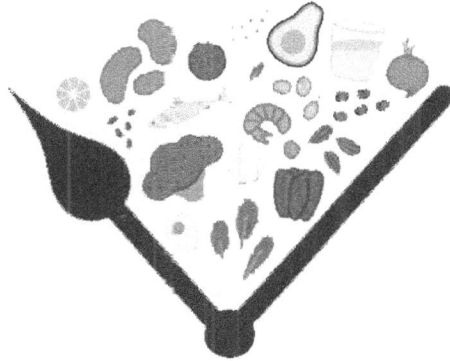

There are different types or methods of intermittent fasting that can be quite effective. The trick is finding out which is the best one for you that suits your needs and lifestyle.

## The More Popular Types of Intermittent Fasting Methods

Fasting has periods where you do not eat and then periods called cycles, patterns, or eating windows where a person can eat. The following methods are the most effective for weight loss and are the easiest fasting cycles to follow.

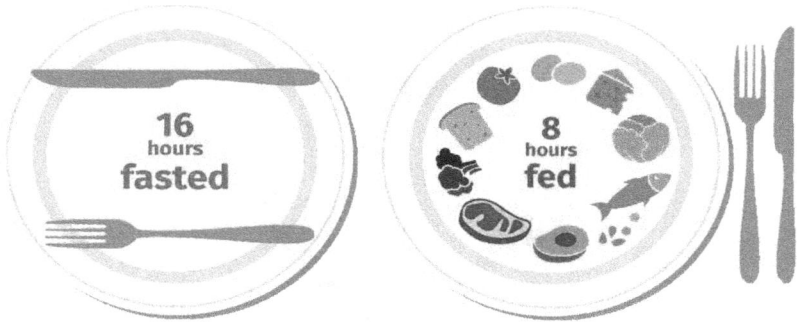

The 16:8 intermittent fasting method is also known as the 8-hour diet as you fast for 16-hours a day and have an 8-hour a day eating window. This method is used by a lot of celebrities and top business people as well as being a popular trending diet on social media.

It is used to help lower the risk of contracting a chronic disease, aids in weight loss, and helps with mental acuity. There is a risk with this type of diet as well as it can lead to overeating within the limited time window if a person does not eat correctly. This is because there is no actual diet or restrictions on what you eat or how much you eat during that time window.

During the 16-hours of fasting a person can consume nothing but unsweetened beverages such as water, tea, or coffee. You should not be consuming fizzy drinks, alcohol, or any other sweetened beverages because they are not healthy for you. They can also lead to health problems because of what goes into those kinds of beverages.

During the 8-hour eating windows, a person is free to eat what they please. Most people who do the 16:8 fasting method find it easier to fast during the evening and through breakfast the next day. Leaving their 8-hour eating window to start at around noon or one o'clock. In order to get the full benefits of an intermittent fasting diet, it can be beneficial to follow a diet plan that suits you. A lot of people will follow diets such as the keto meal plan, weight watchers, low-carb diets, and so on.

The diet you choose should be one that is beneficial to you and caters to your eating needs. What you do not want to do when you are trying to reap the benefits of intermittent fasting is to fill yourself up on empty carbs and sweets. Rather make the most out of your eating window and eat healthily.

This intermittent fasting method is not really for beginners and if you would like to try it you should try a modified version of it. Maybe go to 12:12, fast for 12 hours and eat for 12 hours on a healthy eating plan. Only fast with this method no more than twice a week when you first start with intermittent fasting.

## 5:2 Intermittent Fasting Method

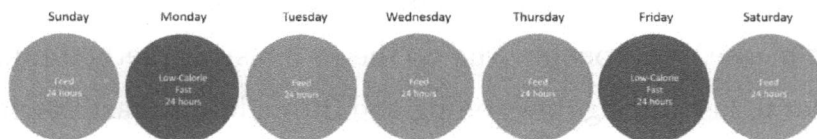

The 5:2 diet is currently the most popular and practiced method of intermittent fasting and is known as the fast diet. Michael Mosley, a British journalist who was diagnosed with type 2 diabetes in 2012 was the one who popularized this method. He managed to turn his life around by losing 26.5 pounds in 12 weeks which helped him get his type 2 diabetes under control.

Throughout our lives, we are told that breakfast is the most important meal of the day. But who says it has to be eaten as soon as we get up or grab something as we rush out the door to start the day? Michael Mosley developed the 5:2 diet believing that a person needs to give their body a rest from food.

The belief of the diet is that when a person goes without food for more than 10-hours the body goes into what is called negative protein or nitrogen balance. When this happens, the body starts to consume and get rid of old proteins and does not produce new ones. When the body does not receive enough or quality protein it starts to consume what it can find and switches the body to cell repair mode.

An early supper and late breakfast are a good way to give the body a chance to completely clean itself out and repair what needs to be repaired. On the 5:2 diet, a person will eat a normal healthy diet for five days of the week. The other two days they will be on a calorie-restricted diet of 500 to 600 calories a day.

A person can choose the two days of the week that best suits them as long as there is at least one to two days in between fasting days. For instance, fast on a Tuesday, eat the normal number of calories required on Wednesday, then fast on Thursday or Friday again. On fasting days, a woman should consume around 500 calories and try to have two small meals for the day. The best eating plan is to have a late breakfast and an early supper to get the best results.

On eating days, a proper, healthy diet should be followed in order to lose weight and enjoy other health benefits of the diet along with regular exercise.

## Alternate Day Fasting (ADF) Method

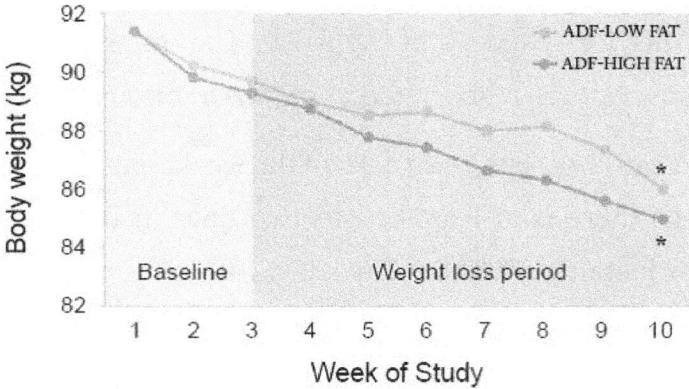

Alternate day fasting or ADF is a fasting method done over a 48-hour period. A person will fast for 36-hours (a day and a half) then eat normally for the 12-hour eating window. Of course, non-sweetened beverages such as water, tea, and coffee with no sugar can be drunk but nothing else during the 36-hours.

During the 12-hour eating window, people can eat a healthy normal diet or anything they want. There is a more popular version of this fasting method where people eat within a certain time period and may consume up to 500 calories. Dr. Krista Varady brought out the "Every Other Day Diet" after studying the alternate-day fasting method.

Beginners to fasting methods find this intermittent fasting diet to be the easiest to maintain. There have been some studies that show this method to be most effective for middle-aged women in losing and controlling their weight. Other studies have shown that it may be able to reduce inflammation markers as well as belly fat in for those who are obese.

The alternate-day fasting method has shown to work with or without a low-fat diet but is most effective when combined with regular exercise. In order to stop or reduce compensatory hunger, the modified version of this fasting method is the most recommended. Eating 500 calories a day at a certain time on fasting days with this method reduces hunger.

### Eat Stop Eat Intermittent Fasting Method

Brad Pilon developed this method of fasting after doing research on how it affects metabolism. The eat stop eat method of fasting became popular after he wrote his popular book, *Eat Stop Eat*.

This fasting method requires a person to have two days a week when they fast. These days must not be consecutive days though and should have at least one to two eating days in between.

It sounds a bit painful as a person has to commit to fast for a full 24-hours. For instance, a person could choose Monday and Thursday as their fasting days. This ensures that there are two full days in between their fasting days. Choose time to start fasting from Monday which could be at 10 am which gives you time to eat a good breakfast before beginning your fast.

The fast would then end at 10 am on Tuesday where a person can indulge in a good breakfast. They would eat their normal diet from 10 am Tuesday until 10 am Thursday when they would start to fast again. The fast would stop at 10 am Friday and for the rest of the weekend, the person gets to eat their normal diet.

Although there are no actual dietary requirements for non-fasting days, it is highly recommended to follow a healthy diet. Or at least make healthy food choices and choose foods that have slow-releasing carbs to eat just before starting the fast.

No matter what fasting method a person chooses, it is imperative that they keep themselves well hydrated. Water is always the best solution although an unsweetened coffee or tea can be a nice change.

### The Warrior Diet

The warrior diet is quite a strict intermittent fasting method as it follows a 20-hour restricted calorie intake diet and a 4-hour unrestricted diet window per day. This diet is based on the habits of human ancestors that would go hunting and gathering during the day. This would be for most of the day starting in the early hours of the morning to return when the sun was going down. It was during these few hours before they slept that they would eat.

The warrior diet is based on fasting during the night and into the next day until dinner time. Then for 4-hours it is recommended that a person eats nutrient-dense foods although there is no actual limit to what a person can eat during this window. It is, however, advisable to eat good foods such as lots of whole-foods. Unprocessed foods are the foods to aim for on this diet and the good news is you don't have to count calories for 4-hours.

### One Meal a Day (OMAD) Diet

This is not the fasting method recommended for beginners and it should not be taken lightly. Before going on this diet, a person should first check with their medical advisor as it is a 23:1 fasting method. This means that a person cannot consume any calories for 23 hours of the day and only has a 1-hour eating window in which to eat.

Before trying this fasting method, a person should learn the best times of day to eat. They should also learn what the best foods are to eat within the 1-hour eating window. They should also only do it once or at most twice a week unless they really know what they are doing.

It does, however, offer rapid weight loss and is not too hard to follow. There is also no need for calories to be counted on the diet. In the 1-hour eating window, a person can eat any food they want. Once again healthy food choices are always the best option.

# Chapter 3: The Benefits of Fasting for Women Over 50

Studies have shown that intermittent fasting may be extremely useful for postmenopausal women to aid in maintaining their weight. There are quite a few benefits to intermittent fasting for middle-aged women or women that are going through menopause no matter their age.

#1:
Fat Loss

#2:
Improved
Cognitive Function

#3:
Lower
Inflammation

#4:
Lower Blood
Pressure

#5:
Blood Sugar
Control

#6:
Better Metabolic
Health

#7:
Longevity

## Why for Women Over 50?

Women who approach post-menopause (and sometimes even as early as pre-menopause) tend to start accumulating belly fat. They will start noticing their metabolism get slower. They may also start feeling aches and pains in their joints. Their sleep patterns start to get completely out of routine leaving them feeling exhausted all the time. Then there is the weight gain and also a higher risk of developing chronic diseases like cancer, diabetes, and heart disease that could lead to heart attacks.

There is also the risk of neurodegenerative diseases, stroke, and a constant feeling of fatigue. Intermittent fasting has been known to reset a person's internal balance. This, in turn, boosts their external appearance, energy levels, and cuts down on stress as they control their weight.

## Why Should Women Choose the Intermittent Fasting Diet?

Intermittent fasting has become a very popular healthy lifestyle trend, and for good reason. It offers many health benefits as well as improves a person's state of mind and encourages an all-round feeling of well-being.

# Benefits of Intermittent Fasting for Women Over 50

## INCREASES

- The intensity of the fat burning stage for Keto adapters
- Leptin levels to reduce overeating
- Insulin and leptin sensitivity (lowers risk of cancer, heart disease, and diabetes)

## DECREASES

- Weight gain and metabolic damage
- Inflammation and oxidative stress
- Reduces insulin resistance
- Cholesterol levels
- Speed of aging process

When women get to 50 and over, their skin will start to show signs of age. They may find their joints start to ache for no reason, and suddenly belly fat accumulates as if you have just given birth. There are so many creams, diets and exercises on the market to tighten the skin and try to help. The fact is, they may work to a certain point but then the body hits a shelf, and nothing seems to push a person past it. This boils up frustration making women look into the more drastic and very expensive alternatives like surgery. Which in itself poses so many more dangers and risks for women of 50 and over.

A person does not need to go under the knife or starve themselves to reboot their system or change their shape. Intermittent fasting is a much cheaper and less risky way to do this and there is no need to make any drastic eating habit changes either. Well, you may need to make a few adjustments like cutting out junk food and eating healthier. But once again the diet a person follows is their personal choice and depends on how serious they are about becoming healthier.

Some health benefits of intermittent fasting for women over 50 include:

## *Activating Cellular Repair*

Fasting has been known to kick start the body's natural cellular repair function, get rid of mature cells, improve longevity, and improve hormone function. All things that tend to take a battering as people age. This can alleviate joint and muscle aches as well as lower back pain. As the cells are being repaired and damage undone, it helps with the skin's elasticity and health too.

## *Increase Cognitive Function and Protects the Brain from Damage*

Intermittent fasting may increase the levels of a brain hormone known as a brain-derived neurotrophic factor (BDNF). It may equally guard the brain against damage like a stroke or Alzheimer's disease as it promotes new nerve cell growth. It also increases cognitive function and could effectively defend a person against other neurodegenerative diseases as well.

## Weight Loss

When people have belly fat, it can cause many health problems that are associated with various diseases as it indicates a person has visceral fat. Visceral fat is fat that goes deep into the abdominal surrounding the organs. Belly fat is terribly hard to lose, especially for an aging woman. Intermittent fasting has been known to help reduce not only weight but inches of over five percent of body fat in around twenty-two to twenty-five weeks (Barna, 2019).

## Alleviates Oxidative Stress and Inflammation

Oxidative stress is when the body has an imbalance of antioxidants as well as free radicals. This imbalance can cause both tissue and cell damage in overweight as well as aging people. It can also lead to various chronic illnesses like cancer, heart disease, diabetes, and also has an impact on the signs of aging. Oxidative stress can trigger the inflammation that causes these diseases.

Intermittent fasting can provide your system with a reboot, helping to alleviate oxidative stress and inflammation in a middle-aged woman. It also significantly reduces the risk of oxidative stress and inflammation for those overweight or obese.

## Slow Down the Aging Process

As intermittent fasting gives both the metabolism and cellular repair a reboot it offers the potential to slow down aging. It may even prolong a person's lifespan by quite a few years especially if following a nutritious diet and exercise regime alongside intermittent fasting.

# Chapter 4: Balancing Hormones and Boosting Energy

The endocrine system is the body's system that produces hormones. Hormones are potent chemicals that convey messages through the body to regulate certain processes. Hormones are needed for growth, fertility, metabolism, the immune system, and a person's mood or behavior.

## Hormones

As we age our hormones change and our body produces more of some, less of others. Hormones are produced in accordance with the person's stage of life. For example, a teenager's hormones are produced to get them through puberty. The following stage of development for the human body where hair starts to develop in strategic places. A woman's body changes and starts to get ready for the subsequent stage, which is to produce offspring.

During pregnancy, the body produces the human chorionic gonadotropin (HCG) hormone. As well as human placental lactogen (HPL) hormone, estrogen, and progesterone. As most people know, women seem all over the place both physically and emotionally when they are expecting. Now you know why with all these extremely potent chemicals being produced.

Women go through perimenopause usually during their mid-forties. At this stage, the body's estrogen production starts to slow down until they go through menopause. During menopause, the body stops releasing eggs which means a woman is no longer able to reproduce.

Most women will go through menopause between the ages of fifty-one to fifty-two. It can last anywhere from one to three years and the symptoms of menopause can include:

- The menstrual cycle has stopped for a year or more.
- Problems sleeping.
- Bad night sweats that can drench a person.
- Uncomfortably dry or itchy skin that actually feels like you have a thousand ants crawling on you.
- Problems with urination like releasing little drops when sneezing, problems urinating, and incontinence issues.
- Urinary tract infections or dryness which leaves a burning sensation.
- Decreased libido and disinterest in intimacy.
- Some women experience varying degrees of lethargy.
- Hot flashes that cause a person to feel like the doors of hell have opened in front of them. These come on suddenly with no warning at any time or place during the day.

Some women will experience all of these symptoms, some of them, and others may get them more mildly or not at all. Menopause and its symptoms are a lot like being pregnant without giving birth at the end. The hormones or lack thereof, affect each woman differently. It wholly depends on how your body adjusts to the current phase in its lifecycle.

It is vital to try and balance your hormones. One hormone which increases when practicing intermittent fasting is the growth hormone. As soon as a person stops eating for long enough, the body starts to produce this hormone. It is the hormone sent out to repair tissue and is typically called the fountain of youth hormone due to its reparative qualities. While it doesn't do much to change menopause, it will help slow down the aging process and help you retain muscle. It also helps with weight loss, and intermittent fasting has been shown to almost double this hormone in the body.

During menopause, two hormones that become imbalanced are melatonin and cortisol. These are the hormones that need to be in sync, as melatonin helps a person sleep and enjoy good quality sleep. While cortisol is the hormone that helps a person wake up, feel alert, and keep the mind clear. An imbalance of these two hormones is usually due to a health problem, anxiety, stress, and menopause. Intermittent fasting along with proper nutrition may aid in the production and balance of these two hormones.

Homeostasis is the term used for hormone balance and it is vital for optimum health. To be successful with an intermittent fasting program, you also need a nutritious diet. Once a woman reaches fifty it is imperative to live a healthy lifestyle to ensure you enjoy your golden years in peak form.

Women over fifty should strive to:

- Eat well but healthily and make smarter food choices.
- Fast within their comfort zone and make it a part of their life.
- Take supplements to ensure they are getting enough vitamins and minerals.
- Take care of their skin by implementing the proper treatments in or out of the sun.
- Wear protection in the heat when outside. Wear a hat to cover your face and neck. Wear sun protection, although a good 15 minutes of direct sunlight will increase vitamin D.
- Exercise at least two to three times a week, more if you are able to.
- Most importantly drink lots of water.

## Energy

Hormones can equally affect a person's energy levels. During menstrual cycles, energy levels have been known to spike and rise due to increased levels of estrogen. But after the menstrual cycle, the levels of estrogen drop quite drastically causing lethargy. As women reach menopause and estrogen levels start to drop, women feel less energetic and extremely tired.

Another hormonal culprit that contributes to a menopausal woman's lack of energy is progesterone. This hormone declines with age and is one of the reasons middle-aged women have problems sleeping. Progesterone is used to induce ovulation in younger women, but it also promotes sleep. Obviously, a woman going through middle age no longer has need of ovulation, so her body does not produce as much as it used to.

Although they do not produce it in the amounts a man does, a woman's body also produces testosterone. Testosterone performs a significant part in the production of red blood cells in the body. Red blood cells are the cells that transport oxygen around the body which is a much-needed component in the promotion of energy. As with many other hormones, menopause limits the production of testosterone as well.

High-stress levels will cause an increase in cortisol, which as discussed in the previous section, you will know keeps a person awake. This affects sleep patterns, which is just another added factor causing a lack of energy due to feeling tired. It will also have an impact on a woman's mood and leave them feeling horrible.

There are ways to increase energy levels but the first step to take is to measure your hormone levels. This can be done by your medical advisor, a registered clinic, or there are home tests you can buy at the drugstore. Ask a pharmacist what the best and most reliable brands are. Once you know what you are dealing with there are a few methods you can try to increase energy levels.

Never try hormone replacements or balancing hormones without the advice of a medical professional. If you are not on any medication or have any pre-existing medical conditions you can try one of the following tips:

- Ask your doctor, nutritionist, or pharmacist to recommend a good quality multi-vitamin. Make sure you fall into a routine of taking them.
- Slowly change your diet to one that offers more nutrition and agrees with your system. As you age you will find foods that you may no longer be able to eat.
- Find a quiet time to take ten to fifteen minutes to meditate, clear your mind, and learn the art of breathing. Tibetan monks have practiced *anapanasati,* which is mindfulness through breathing.
- Get enough good quality sleep. You may need to make some adjustments to your bedroom. Make sure your pillow is supporting your head and that your mattress is doing the same for your body. Take all electronics out of your room, if you use your mobile phone for an alarm make sure it goes into sleep mode. Instead of a TV, make room for a chair to curl up in and read. Reading before bed is a great way to unwind and slip into another world to clear your mind. Try not taking naps during the day.
- Get in some exercise at least once a day, twice if you can manage it. It does not mean you have to go running a marathon or do the Tour de France. Go for a walk, do

some gardening, or take a gentle bike ride and look at the scenery.

- Find a new hobby or take up an old one you had put aside. If you engage your mind, you will automatically gear your body up for action.

- There are supplements and certain foods to naturally boost your energy. Whatever you do, do not try highly caffeinated drinks, or other such types of energy boosters you find in a supermarket.

By now you will know the next bit of advice is going to be — drink lots of water. It is a great cure for a whole lot of things including lethargy. If you want to get a little extra boost, try using an icepack on your Vagus nerve in your neck for a minute at a time.

# Chapter 5: Definitive Weight Loss and Increased Mental Clarity

Clean eating, movement, breathing, and fasting have been known to stimulate weight loss as well as clear the mind.

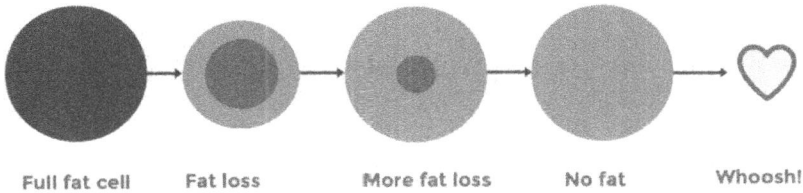

Full fat cell     Fat loss     More fat loss     No fat     Whoosh!

## Weight Loss

Losing weight is a mindset really. You have to be motivated to want it and be prepared to do it. Like anything else in life, you have to be mentally prepared for it and want it badly enough to follow through. There are many roadblocks in life and one of the biggest we have to overcome are our own mental roadblocks.

One of the biggest things that hold us back is fear, even if we do not realize we actually fear something. Actual fear is easier to overcome as more often than not we know it is some ingrown irrational state of mind that makes us fear. Like a fear of heights may be a fear of falling from that height and not the actual height itself.

Instead of working our way through it, we simply avoid it, or cower somewhere in the middle of a crowd and peek out at the amazing world from above. It is easy to hide from our fears these days. As the internet allows us to travel, get to the top of the highest mountain, or be who we want to be. We can do all this safely through our screens where we know we have nothing to fear.

Losing weight, getting fit, and being healthy is no different. Before the internet, a person would have to go out and research things like fasting. You actually had to face a person, look them in the eye and have them assess you.

Most fasting for weight loss programs would need to be done through a trained professional. These days all the information you want is on the internet at your fingertips. You can gather it, do all the leg work, and sort out your way forward. The trick is, to have the fortitude to actually start the program and stick with it to reach your goals.

Unlike a monitored weight-loss and fast program, the only person monitoring your program is you. So you have to be both the antagonist and protagonist of your new lifestyle change. You are the one that will need to motivate, monitor, and maintain your program. There is not going to be any gold stars or pats on the back when you do reach your targets.

What you will have instead is a feeling of accomplishment along with starting to feel and look great. You have to be happy with that and realize the only one you need to impress is you. The only one benefiting from your new lifestyle change is going to be you. The only one who can push you through this and get you to where you want to go is you.

Even people who go on a monitored program need to realize that at the end of the day this is all about and for them. The professionals are not getting anything out of it, except maybe money and another client reference. It is their job, but this is your life, your wellbeing, and your quality of life.

Self-help books, trained and qualified professionals, support groups, and family can only get you to a certain point. It is like going up to the top of the tallest building fearing heights. Why go up there if you are unwilling to take that one small step that will allow you to see for miles around you? Until you are willing to try and take that step there really is no point in going up there. Just like intermittent fasting and clean eating, if you are unwilling to take that first step and commit, you are not going to get anywhere.

Doing all the groundwork to gear yourself up to start with fasting and a new diet is like taking that long ride up to the top of the building. You may think, "I will do it next time" or "I will start tomorrow". But what if next time or tomorrow is too late?

Procrastination is a person's worst enemy and leads to the inevitable if only statement. 'If only' does not help anyone and leads to depression, low self-esteem, and regret. But 'wow look at me now' energy leads to high spirits, high self-esteem, confidence-filled energy and vitality. It is taking that chance to step forward and trust that you will not fall only to be rewarded with breathtaking scenery and a feeling of triumph.

Can do and will do attitudes are the way to success. Losing weight and fasting are mostly a mindset, get yours in the correct set to achieve your goals.

Make yourself want to try new food groups, get excited about trying something new. Think about how you feel after a good scrub in the shower or day at the spa. How clean, shiny, and new you feel. When you go shopping for food or order from a restaurant or look at dinner menus think about feeling clean on the inside.

## Mental Clarity

Fasting helps with mental clarity as it gives the body time to clean itself out and do a lot of reparative housework. Housework is hard to do when the body has to continually digest food from morning through to the evening.

Starting to fast, as with starting anything new, is hard and takes a lot of discipline as well as committed dedication. Most people who have trained their entire lives and stuck to healthy lifestyles may be able to make the adjustment to fasting more quickly.

But like dieting it is a mental transition. One of the best ways to make the transition is to start off with an activity that balances as well as centers a person. Some good examples of finding balance are meditation, the art of breathing, and exercises like yoga or tai chi.

### *Mindfulness Meditation*

There have been studies that show meditation may be beneficial to one's mental and physical health. Mindfulness comes in when a person becomes aware of everything around them and is present in the moment without becoming stressed or overwhelmed.

Even though every human being on the planet has the ability to be mindful we do not all practice it on a daily basis. If you think of someone who is experienced in a trained discipline like martial arts. They learn to use their senses to be mindful of all those around them. They train their senses to become alert and can actually sense danger.

Animals in the wild use these senses every minute of their lives to stay alive. As apex predators and having been spoiled by not having to hunt or forage for our food, human beings' senses have been dulled. As a result, most of us have lost touch with more than just the world around us but our inner selves as well.

Mindful meditation is meant as a way to re-tune those senses and wake them up. Being mindful may actually rewire the physical structure of a person's brain. Research has shown that over time meditation creates some changes in the grey matter of the brain. In a control study group, participants of a meditation study reported they were less stressed, they felt better able to cope with their daily life after 27-hours of collective meditation over a period of time. (Holzel, Carmody, Vangel, Congleton, Yerramsetti, Gard, Lazar, 2011)

Meditation in itself is a journey we take into our minds. It is learning how to explore the fascinating system that is our body. Understanding its uniqueness, its likes and dislikes, and what it needs. It is a discovery of experiencing the full feeling of our senses, emotions, as well as our thoughts.

Mixing mindfulness in with meditation gives that journey another dimension and forces us to open up more than just what is within us. It helps us experience what is around us as well and how that affects us on a subconscious level.

Once you understand meditation, you will find that you can slip in and out of that state whenever or wherever. Even if it is just for a minute or two to quiet your mind and restore calm. It is within these moments where we can also put into practice mindfulness as we take that moment to concentrate on our breath and surroundings.

Mindful meditation helps a person achieve peace and calm within. It is a good place to start to take the next step towards fasting. It is also where you can reprogram yourself to accept the new lifestyle change and embrace the many benefits it is going to bring.

Fasting and meditation bring a great balance to a person's lifestyle. These practices have been used together for centuries. They have been used by various cultures to purify both the body and the soul. When used together they can become a powerful tool in understanding just how powerful the mind-body connection truly is.

### *Learning To Breathe*

To breathe is done as a reflex, in fact, we are so used to this reflex we hardly pay attention to cur breath. On average a person will take around 23,000 breaths without even realizing it. Well, unless there is a problem or an unappealing smell around us.

Buddhist monks are taught to be aware of their breath as it cultivates physical, mental, and emotional well-being. They use the breath to help them achieve mindfulness, balance and align their focus. Buddha teaches that to attain the Four Establishments of Mindfulness one must first be able to practice mindful breathing.

The four establishments of mindfulness are:

- Being mindful of our body.
- Being mindful of our mind and subconscious.
- Being mindful of our emotions, feelings, and sensations.

- Being mindful of the objects which are in our mind.

Learning to use our breath correctly to center and balance us to mindfulness helps to improve a person's concentration and thus their focus. By becoming aware of our breath, we allow it to flow more freely, we can use it to control stress, pain, and emotions. It can heighten our sensations and establish greater awareness within us and around us.

Learning to use our breath with mindful meditation is one more powerful tool to increase the benefits of intermittent fasting. It is also a way to help ready ourselves to accept and cope with intermittent fasting. Being able to breathe and control our breath also helps with our physical fitness, it can also lift any fog clouding the brain.

If you are feeling fatigued, irritated, or are running out of energy, straighten your diaphragm and practice your breathing. Once you are aware of your breathing, you can start realizing your breathing patterns. For instance, when some people get stressed, they tend to hold in their breath for longer periods of time. When you are anxious or angry, your breathing may become more rapid and your heart rate speeds up.

Knowing how to breathe to get your emotions and body in check is a good way to alleviate stress, anxiety, and lower your blood pressure too.

*Movement*

Mindfulness meditation and breathing can be combined with the gentle art of movement. You can try yoga which helps to strengthen your core, balance, and improves blood flow. It helps to cleanse your mind, body, and soul as energy flows through you.

Tai chi is another discipline that gently exercises the body, clears the mind, practices mindful breathing, and allows energy to flow through you. Tai chi is good for improving posture, improving physical balance, increasing muscle strength, and mobility. It is so gentle it can be practiced well into advanced years.

## Putting It All Together

If you start off with one of the above techniques and stick to it. It will seem like a natural progression to the next stage which would be to start intermittent fasting. Once you start to feel the benefits of fasting, mindful meditation, breathing, and movement you will want to eat healthily.

Building yourself up for success is better done in stages than just jumping in feet first. You are establishing a new way of life one section at a time. Adapting and modifying one part of the process before moving onto the next process until you have reached your goal.

# Chapter 6: What You Need to Know

There are a few things that a person needs to know before diving in and proceeding with intermittent fasting. One of the first things is that it may be a good idea to have a general checkup and chat with your medical practitioner before you start fasting. A few blood workups or a complete physical can establish a baseline from which to begin. You will be able to figure out an ideal fasting plan as well as a suitable diet that includes any supplements, micronutrients, and macronutrients you may require.

## Why the Intermittent Fasting Diet is More Than Just Weight Loss

The intermittent fasting diet is more than just a diet. It is a lifestyle choice. When you put the word diet on anything it automatically causes a mental block. That is a person's first stumbling block and one that can be removed easily enough. Rather think about intermittent fasting as making a lifestyle choice to improve your physical, mental, and overall health. The weight loss that may come with it, is an added bonus. It will also boost your self-esteem and energy levels which will in themselves greatly improve the quality of your life.

Intermittent fasting offers all the health benefits already discussed in this book along with learning self-control which leads to self-discipline. It offers mental clarity and puts you in tune with your body as you learn to differentiate between real hunger and that phantom hunger that demands satisfaction. Intermittent fasting makes you feel refreshed, clean and energized from the inside out. It is not a feeling you can gain from exercise, detoxing, or leading a healthy lifestyle it can only be felt after a bout of fasting.

You sleep better, heal better, feel better, have more energy, and as your mind is not foggy you are able to think on your feet. As a result, your stress levels decrease as anxiety starts to wane, and you feel more like a whole person again. But as with everything in life, it does come with warnings as we have stressed numerous times throughout the book. Intermittent fasting may not be for everyone and, depending on your health, you may need a modified version of one of the fasting methods.

## What You Need to Know About Intermittent Fasting

Until you are well trained in intermittent fasting you should make yourself a schedule of your fasting days and times. The most straightforward intermittent fasting method to start on is the 5:2 method. In this method, you eat normally for 5 days of the week and then fast for the other 2 days. You will need to pick the two days of the week that will best suit you, making sure there is at least one to two days between fasting days.

During the two fasting days of the week, as a woman, you should consume no more than 500 calories a day. You can consume beverages that contain no calories as already discussed. Beverages like tea, coffee, and water with no added sweeteners. Water is always the best option as it makes you feel full and is an excellent source of hydration

## *Fasting Plan for 5:2 Combined With 12:12*

When you are first starting out you may want to have a four-week cycle.

For instance:

### **Week 1**

Fasting Days are Monday and Thursday. Fasting time is 12 hours with only non-caloric beverages and 12 hours where you can eat a maximum of 500 calories per day (two meals).

For Monday start fasting at 9 pm on Sunday night after you have had a good filling supper and stop fasting at 9 am Monday Morning until 9 pm on Monday night. Have an unsweetened coffee or tea for breakfast at 9 am, lunch to a total of 250 calories at 1 pm, and then supper at 7 or 8 pm of 250 calories. Tuesday morning you can start eating normally for the day.

For Thursday start fasting at 9 pm on Wednesday night after you have enjoyed a nice hearty supper. Follow the same fasting regiment as above and eat normally from Friday.

**Week 2**

Choose two different weekdays like Tuesday and Friday.

For Tuesday start fasting at 9 pm on Monday night after a hearty supper and follow the same method as Monday/Thursday above. Eat normally on Wednesday and Thursday for the day.

Friday you can start to fast at 9 pm on Thursday night once again after a good supper. Follow the same method as Monday, Thursday, and Tuesday above. You can start eating normally on Saturday morning again.

**Week 3**

Choose another two different days of the week like Wednesday and Saturday. Most people balk at having to fast on a Saturday, but it takes great discipline and you can always keep Sundays as your non-fasting day.

Wednesday you will start fasting at 9 pm on Tuesday night, following the same method as the days above, to start eating normally again on Thursday morning.

Saturday you will start fasting at 9 pm on Friday night. Follow the same method as the days above where you can start eating normally on Sunday morning.

## Week 4

On week 4 you should not fast but instead eat normally every day then start the fasting week over the next week again.

## Non-Fasting Days

As with the methods above, the days where you are not fasting you will eat a normal diet. Although there are no specific diet rules to follow when you are on eating days, or eating windows, it is highly recommended to follow a good, nutritious diet. After all, you want to reap the full benefits of this way of life, see results, and feel better. You may still reap some of the benefits if you eat what you like.

To make life even easier for you, find out what your recommended daily calorie intake is. This is determined by your height, bone structure, muscle mass, the way you carry your fat deposits, as well as your age and gender.

Once you have that you can find out what your weekly calorie intake should be.

For example, an average woman needs 2,000 calories a day to maintain a healthy weight, fasting days are 25% of the 2,000 calories (500 calories).

2,000 calories per day x 7 days = 14,000 calories a week

500 calories per day x 2 fasting days = 1,000 calories a week for fasting days

14,000 calories per week - 1,000 calories a week for fasting days = 13,000 calories a week

13,000 calories per week / 5 non-fasting days per week = 2,800 calories per non-fasting days

You should eat within your weekly calorie amount and not go over. It is better to try and keep your calories either at 14,000 calories per week and 2,000 calories per non-fasting days. To really boost your metabolism, try calorie cycling with your non-fasting days. Calories cycling is when you eat 2,000 calories one day, 1,000 calories another day, then 2,250 calories on another day, non-fasting days that is.

When calorie cycling you must not exceed your weekly calorie amount. If you start your calorie cycling on a Monday, then you only have until that Sunday night to eat your weekly amount. The following Monday your calories set back to 14,000 calories.

Choose a good diet or make healthy food choices if you are going to continue with your normal eating patterns. You do not have to make drastic changes but instead of reaching for a treat full of empty carbs reach for one that has some nutritional value. They are not loaded with anything artificial and taste just as good. Before you know it, you will have retrained your mind to rather opt for the healthier alternative to your favorite foods or beverages.

# 7-Day Intermittent Food Plan

One way to keep on a healthy diet is to plan your meals for the week ahead of time. That way you can get the shopping done more efficiently as you know exactly what you want to buy. It is also a great way to budget. You can prepare some meals in advance to save time, and you keep yourself on a healthy eating track.

## *Food Plan*

The following 7-day meal plan is an example of what you can eat on your fasting days and non-fasting days. Remember to stay within your weekly calorie limit and go for the healthier choices. For instance, instead of taking full-fat vanilla ice cream, choose low-fat and sugar-free. Choose raw almonds instead of salted ones and so on.

### Day 1 — Fasting Day 500 Calorie Allowance

*9:00 AM Breakfast — 0 calories*

A cup of unsweetened coffee or tea.

*1:00 PM Lunch — 231 calories*

1 small baked potato with ½ tsp butter and 2 tsp sour cream topped with ½ tsp chopped fresh chives.

Garden salad with ¼ cup of iceberg lettuce, 1 small celery stalk, 1 medium tomato, and drizzle with 1 tsp of balsamic vinegar.

*8:00 PM Supper — 223 calories*

¼ medium avocado, 1 tsp balsamic vinegar, and 1 slice of whole-wheat toast.

Add the same garden salad as above and add ¼ cucumber.

## Day 2 — Non-Fasting Day 2 000 Calorie Allowance

*9:00 AM Breakfast — 412 calories*

2-egg omelet with 2 tbsp cheddar cheese, 1 tsp chopped spring onion, and 1 tbsp chopped button mushrooms.

1 slice of whole wheat toast with 1 tsp butter.

*11:00 AM Snack — 166 calories*

½ cup low-fat Greek yogurt, with 1 tsp organic honey, and ½ cup halved strawberries (fresh or frozen).

*1:00 PM Lunch — 491 calories*

6 shoots of grilled asparagus and 1 salmon fillet with lemon butter and dill sauce.

1 bowl of Caesar salad with dressing and croutons.

1 cup sugar-free butterscotch pudding.

*3:00 PM Snack — 150 calories*

 2 tbsp feta cheese, ¼ cup of olives, 2 tbsp low-fat cottage cheese, 3 small breadsticks.

*8:00 PM Supper — 698 calories*

1 flame-grilled cheeseburger with a 1 cup of oven-baked fries with low-sodium salt to taste.

1 cup fat-free vanilla ice cream with ½ cup blueberries (fresh or frozen) and ½ cup raspberries (fresh or frozen).

*10:00 PM Snack — 66 calories*

½ cup of blackberries and 5 raw almonds.

## Day 3 — Non-Fasting Day 2 000 Calorie Allowance

*9:00 AM Breakfast — 492 calories*

1 cup of organic rolled oats cooked, add ¼ cup unsweetened almond milk, 1 sliced banana, ¼ cup mixed berries (frozen or fresh), 3 tsp organic honey, and 2 tbsp raw almond slices.

*11:00 AM Snack — 128 calories*

½ cup low-fat plain chunky cottage cheese with 2 tsp organic honey, 2 tbsp blackberries, 2 tbsp raspberries, and 1 tbsp raw cashew nuts. The berries can be either fresh or frozen and the cashews should be unsalted.

*1:00 PM Lunch — 393 calories*

2 slices whole wheat bread, 2 tsp butter, 2 slices of turkey, 2 tbsp shredded cheddar cheese, 1 tsp low-fat mayonnaise, ¼ sliced tomato, 2 lettuce leaves, and 2 tsp alfalfa sprouts. Make a delicious filling sandwich.

Slice up ¼ apple, 5 grapes, 2 tbsp low-fat Greek yogurt, 1 tsp organic honey, ¼ tsp ground cinnamon, and ¼ tsp cayenne pepper for extra zing (optional). Mix together in a dessert bowl for a treat after your sandwich.

*3:00 PM Snack — 173 calories*

2 plain, no salt added rice cakes, 2 tbsp plain low-fat cream cheese, 1 tsp organic honey, and ¼ tsp ground cinnamon. Spread a bit of cream cheese on each rice cake, drizzle with a bit of the honey and add a dash of ground cinnamon on top.

*8:00 PM Supper — 692 calories*

1 lean grilled chicken breast (spiced as you require and cut into chunks), ¼ cup cooked wild rice, ¼ tsp ground ginger, ¼ tsp ground cinnamon, ¼ cup cooked garden peas, 3 tbsp diced spring onions, and 1 tbsp low-fat mayonnaise. Serve the chicken and rice warm, add the rest of the ingredients after you have mixed up the rice and chicken in a dinner bowl.

1 cup fat-free vanilla ice cream with ½ cup fresh, halved strawberries, 1 diced kiwi, and ½ cup diced fresh mango. Drizzle with 1 tsp organic honey and sprinkle with all-spice as well as chopped raw cashews.

*10:00 PM Snack — 139 calories*

20 raw almonds.

## Day 4 — Fasting Day 500 Calorie Allowance

*9:00 AM Breakfast — 0 calories*

A cup of unsweetened coffee or tea.

*1:00 PM Lunch — 269 calories*

2 large bell peppers (cut in half), 3 tbsp cooked wild rice, 1 tsp capers, ½ oz lean grilled chicken breasts shredded, and 2 tsp

reduced-fat mayonnaise. Divide filling and stuff evenly between each bell pepper half.

*8:00 PM Supper — 224 calories*

1 grilled sole fillet with 1 tsp garlic butter.

Garden salad with 1 cup of iceberg lettuce, 1 medium tomato chopped, ¼ cucumber, 1 tbsp spring onions, ½ cup button mushrooms, 2 tbsp yellow bell pepper, and 1 tbsp organic balsamic vinegar.

## Day 5 — Non-Fasting Day 2 000 Calorie Allowance

*9:00 AM Breakfast — 528 calories*

2 eggs scrambled with 2 tbsp shredded cheddar cheese, 2 tbsp shredded mozzarella cheese, and 1 tsp chopped spring onion.

2 slice of whole wheat toast with 1 tsp butter

1 medium apple

*11:00 AM Snack — 173 calories*

¼ cup regular trail mix

*1:00 PM Lunch — 523 calories*

1 low-carb whole wheat tortilla stuffed with shredded lettuce, ½ chopped tomato, 4 cooked and crumbled pieces of bacon, ¼ chopped avocado, 2 chopped pickles, 1 tbsp low-fat mayonnaise.

1 medium-sized peach

*3:00 PM Snack — 118 calories*

Mixed berry smoothie, 2 tbsp blueberries, 2 tbsp blackberries, 2 tbsp raspberries, ¼ cup organic low-fat unsweetened almond milk, and 4 tbsp low-fat Greek yogurt.

*8:00 PM Supper — 683 calories*

1 large whole wheat tortilla, spread the base with 2 tsp organic unsweetened tomato paste, top with 4 tbsp shredded mozzarella cheese, top with 1 cup cooked shredded chicken breast, ½ thinly sliced tomato. Then top with ½ tsp capers, 1 tbsp pitted black olives, drizzle with 2 tbsp fruit chutney, and last sprinkle 4 tbsp shredded cheddar cheese over the top. Pop the tortilla pizza into a preheated oven and cook for around 18 to 20 minutes or until brown and the ingredients are cooked.

1 large banana sliced lengthwise, ¼ cup fat-free vanilla ice cream, ¼ mixed berries fresh or frozen, 1 large plum cut into chunks, ½ pear cut into chunks, and 1 tbsp unsweetened desiccated coconut. Make the ingredients into a banana boat and top with the desiccated coconut.

*10:00 PM Snack — 150 calories*

4 pieces of dark chocolate.

## Day 6 — Non-Fasting Day 2 000 Calorie Allowance

*9:00 AM Breakfast — 348 calories*

In a dessert bowl or parfait glass add 4 tbsp organic sugar-free granola, top with 5 tbsp fat-free strawberry yogurt, top with 1 tbsp blackberries, 1 tbsp raspberries, 1 tbsp blueberries. Then top with 4 tbsp fat-free plain Greek yogurt, drizzle over 1 tsp organic, honey, sprinkle 1 tsp of toasted almond flakes, 1 tsp chia seeds, and 1 tsp unsweetened desiccated coconut.

*11:00 AM Snack — 183 calories*

1 peanut butter protein bar

2 small apricots

*1:00 PM Lunch — 413 calories*

1 bowl of chicken Caesar salad with dressing and croutons

1 large banana

1 cup of grapes

*3:00 PM Snack — 184 calories*

¼ cup of olives

½ cup of fresh cauliflower divided into florets

½ cup carrots cut into sticks

½ cup cucumber cut into sticks

¼ cup tzatziki

*8:00 PM Supper — 653 calories*

1 roasted chicken breast, 4 roast potatoes, ½ cup cooked corn, ½ cup cooked carrots, and ½ cup cooked peas

1 cup fat-free vanilla ice cream topped with 2 tsp organic cocoa powder, 2 tsp organic honey, and 1 tbsp raw unsalted cashews.

*10:00 PM Snack — 150 calories*

4 pieces of dark chocolate.

## Day 7 — Non-Fasting Day 2 000 Calorie Allowance

*9:00 AM Breakfast — 399 calories*

1 chopped apple, 1 chopped plum, ¼ papaya chopped, 1 banana sliced, ¼ cup fresh halved strawberries, ¼ cup blueberries, 1 tsp sunflower seeds, and 2 tbsp low-fat vanilla Greek yogurt.

1 glass unsweetened organic light coconut milk.

*11:00 AM Snack — 150 calories*

4 pieces of dark chocolate.

*1:00 PM Lunch — 657 calories*

1 bowl of chicken soup with 2 slices of whole wheat toast and 2 tsp butter.

1 small green salad.

1 cup sugar-free butterscotch pudding with ½ cup of fat-free vanilla ice cream.

*3:00 PM Snack — 228 calories*

3 graham crackers with 1 tbsp Nutella.

*8:00 PM Supper — 795 calories*

1 grilled chicken burger with a 1 cup of oven-baked fries with low-sodium salt to taste.

1 small green salad.

1 slice of cheesecake, 1 tbsp low-fat unsweetened whipped cream, and 1 tsp macadamia nuts.

*10:00 PM Snack 104 calories*

½ cup of blackberries, ½ cup of raspberries, and ¼ of blueberries.

**7-Day Food Plan Calorie Summary**

Day 1 (fasting day) = 454 calories in total which is 46 calories less than the daily allowance.

Day 2 (normal eating day) = 1 983 calories in total which is 17 calories less than the daily allowance.

Day 3 (normal eating day) = 2 017 calories in total which is 17 calories more than the daily allowance.

Day 4 (fasting day) = 493 calories in total which is 7 calories less than the daily allowance.

Day 5 (normal eating day) = 2 175 calories in total which is 175 calories more than the daily allowance.

Day 6 (normal eating day) = 1 931 calories in total which is 69 calories less than the daily allowance.

Day 7 (normal eating day) = 2 333 calories in total which is 333 calories more than the daily allowance.

Total calories for the week = 11 386 calories which is 2614 calories less than the weekly total.

As you can see by the meal plan that you can eat great meals, with dessert and still come in well under the recommended calorie intake for the week. All you have to do is make healthier food choices when shopping, going out to eat, or at a dinner party.

# Chapter 7: Ideas for Breakfast, Lunch, and Supper

Eating healthy greatly complements your new fasting lifestyle. But you also have to ensure that you are getting enough nutrition in your diets as well.

## Eating Nutritiously for Women Aged 50 and Over

As a woman, your body has certain nutrient needs that must be fulfilled to maintain good health. You can get a good source of these vitamins and minerals through supplements, but nothing beats the more natural way through food sources.

A lot of women tend to fall short of getting in their daily nutritional requirements. Getting in the correct nutritional requirements can also improve your energy levels, mood, and help control weight gain. As your body ages, you need to help keep it functioning correctly with the correct nutrition. It can also help you through menopause and beyond to ensure you have a good quality of life.

When you are fasting, it is really important to get in as much of your daily recommended nutrients as possible. These help the body to produce hormones and energy, keep the skin healthy, promote healthy teeth, hair, nails, and bones.

The RDA (recommended daily allowance) of the vital nutrients for women 50 and over are:

## Calcium - 1,200 mg per day

Calcium is needed for strong bones and healthy teeth. It also aids in regulating the heartbeat and a deficiency of it affects your teeth, bones, and mood. Not getting enough calcium can lead to osteoporosis. This is because the body will start to take calcium from the bones to aid normal cell function.

Foods that are high in calcium include:

- Low-fat, plain Greek yogurt
- Full-cream milk, non-fat milk, 2% milk, or reduced-fat milk (find a variety fortified with vitamin D).
- Cheeses: cheddar, mozzarella, cream cheese, feta, parmesan, and cottage cheese
- Tofu that states it is made with calcium sulfate
- Nut milk
- Soy milk
- Kale, broccoli, Chinese cabbage, and turnips
- Salmon, shrimp, and sardines
- Oranges and figs
- Fortified cereals
- Baked beans or most canned beans

## Iron - 8 mg per day

Iron is an important nutrient the body needs to maintain healthy hair, skin, nails, and hemoglobin. Hemoglobin is the compound that oxygenates the blood. A deficiency of iron can cause anemia which can cause a person to feel weak and lethargic.

Foods that are high in iron include:

- Raisins
- Bell peppers
- Leafy green vegetables like spinach
- Eggs (boiled)
- Cashew nuts
- Potatoes
- Broccoli, peas, and green beans
- Tuna, oysters, sardines, and muscles
- Turkey and chicken
- Liver
- Beef
- Kidney beans, white beans, lentils, and chickpeas
- Tomatoes
- Bread
- Tofu
- Nuts and seeds
- Some dried fruit
- Breakfast cereals
- Dark chocolate

## Magnesium - 400 mg per day

Magnesium is a nutrient needed to help keep bones and teeth healthy. It also aids in ensuring that your nervous systems and muscles work correctly. Magnesium is needed to support proper insulin levels as well as heart health.

Foods that are high in magnesium include:

- Avocado
- Dark chocolate
- Nuts and seeds
- Most fruit especially raspberries, bananas and figs
- Chickpeas, kidney beans, baked beans, and black beans
- Peas, broccoli, cabbage, green beans, asparagus, and artichokes
- Tuna, mackerel, salmon, and sardines
- Bread, oats, and brown rice
- Cacao (raw organic)
- Tofu
- Leafy green vegetables like kale, spinach, and lettuce

## Vitamin A - 700 mcg per day

Vitamin A is a multifunctional vitamin that plays an important role in keeping the internal organs, kidney, lungs, and heart working as they should. It also supports the immune system, reproduction system, and eyesight.

Foods that are high in vitamin A include:

- Liver

- Cod liver oil
- Tuna, mackerel, trout, and salmon
- Butter
- Cheese, especially goat cheese
- Boiled egg
- Sweet potato, butternut squash, and carrots
- Spinach, broccoli, bell pepper, and lettuce
- Melons and grapefruit

## Vitamin C - 75 mg per day

Vitamin C is another vitamin that plays a crucial part in many operations within the body. It aids the immune system, repairs cell tissue, is vital for growth and normal development. It helps the body absorb iron, and sees to the care of bones, teeth, and muscles. It plays an important part in skin health as it helps with the creation of collagen as well as the healing of wounds.

Foods that are high in vitamin C include:

- Oranges
- Clementines
- Grapefruit
- Kiwis
- Pineapple
- Apricots
- Mangos
- Guava
- Strawberries
- Papaya

- Bell peppers
- Kale
- Brussel Sprouts
- Broccoli
- Cauliflower
- Yellow melons
- Chilis

## Vitamin B-6 - 1.5 mg per day

The B vitamins work together to help with the metabolism, growth, liver function, and the creation of blood cells. Vitamin B-6 is used in the production of the sleep hormone, melatonin.

Foods that are high in vitamin B-6 include:

- Peanuts
- Eggs
- Fish
- Poultry
- Pork
- Bread
- Wholegrain cereals
- Fortified cereals
- Potatoes
- Milk
- Vegetables
- Soya beans

## Vitamin B-9 (Folate) - 400 mcg per day

The B vitamins work together and with other nutrients to create red blood cells. Folate is also an important vitamin that ensures iron is properly absorbed and used in the body. Vitamin B-9 is used to aid in regulating the amino acid homocysteine blood levels.

Foods that are high in vitamin B-9 include:

- Seafood
- Eggs
- Most fresh fruit
- Most fresh fruit juices
- Liver
- Peanuts
- Beans
- Whole grains
- Sunflower seeds
- Broccoli
- Turnip greens
- Asparagus
- Spinach
- Brussel sprouts
- Lettuce
- Green beans

## Vitamin B-12 - 2.4 mcg per day

Vitamin B-12 helps to prevent anemia as it aids the body in properly absorbing and utilizing iron. It helps in the production of DNA and regulates the blood cells and the nervous system.

Foods that are high in vitamin B-12 include:

- Kidneys
- Liver
- Beef
- Other edible animal organs
- Sardines, tuna, trout, herring, and salmon
- Clams, shrimp, mussels, crab, and oysters
- Fortified dairy products
- Eggs
- Ham and pork
- Chicken and turkey
- Plain Greek yogurt
- Cottage, cream cheese, ricotta and mozzarella cheese
- Nutritional yeast

## Vitamin D - 15 mg per day

One of the main functions of vitamin D is helping the body to absorb calcium to ensure healthy bones and teeth. It also supports the immune system, promotes good skin health, may reduce depression, and it can increase weight loss.

Foods that are high in vitamin D include:

- Some nuts and seeds contain vitamin D

- Beef liver
- Egg yolk
- Tuna, salmon, and mackerel
- Fortified dairy products
- Fortified cereals

**Vitamin E — 15 mcg per day**

Vitamin E is like the soldier nutrient of the body. It is used to help fight off harmful bacteria, protects cells against damage, it is an antioxidant, and it boosts the immune system. Vitamin E is also vital for firmer, younger-looking skin.

Foods that are high in vitamin E include:

- Almonds
- Pine nuts
- Peanuts
- Seeds like sunflower seeds
- Spinach
- Broccoli
- Butternut squash
- Avocado
- Kiwi
- Mangos
- Shrimp
- Lobster
- Trout, salmon, and cod
- Goose
- Olive oil

**Vitamin K - 90 mcg per day**

Vitamin K is an important nutrient that helps with bone metabolism and controls calcium levels in the blood. It is also a very important agent that helps in the production of prothrombin which is a protein used in blood clotting.

Foods that are high in vitamin K include:

- Swiss chard
- Mustard greens
- Kale
- Spinach and broccoli
- Liver
- Prunes
- Kiwi
- Hard cheeses
- Avocado
- Green peas
- Cabbage
- Broccoli

## Healthy Eating Ideas

While fasting you should try to eat breakfast later in the day if you are fasting through the night.

If you have chosen the fasting meal plan that allows a person to consume a limited number of calories per day, try to eat only two meals a day — lunch and supper. But if you must eat breakfast then make it a smaller one, take no more than 50 calories from lunch and 70 from dinner. It is better to keep the evening meal lighter than your afternoon one as you need the energy from lunch to get you through the entire day.

### Fasting Plan Without Calorie Restriction

Drink a lot of water which may be infused with mint. Mint keeps you alert and gives the water a nice flavor, but you cannot put anything to sweeten it in the water.

Drink tea or coffee with no sweeteners, sugar, cream, or flavors. You may put a dash of cayenne pepper in the drink to give it a kick and help burn calories.

### Fasting Plan With Calorie Restriction

Fasting day with calorie-restrictive eating windows is based on 500 calories a day.

The breakdown for 500 calories fasting day restriction would be:

With a small breakfast

- Breakfast = 130 calories
- Lunch = 200 calories
- Dinner = 170 calories

Lunch and dinner only

- Breakfast = 0 calories
- Lunch = 250 calories
- Dinner = 250 calories

## *Normal Eating (Non-Fasting) Days or Eating Window Food Ideas*

Non-fasting day food ideas are based on an average of 2,000 calories a day. If you are wanting to lose weight you should look at cutting that down to around 1,500 calories a day.

The breakdown for normal day eating at 2,000 calories a day (14,000 calories per week) would be:

- Breakfast = 500 calories
- Mid-morning snack = 200 calories
- Lunch = 500 calories
- Mid-afternoon snack = 200 calories
- Dinner = 500 calories
- Light before bed snack = 100 calories

Always drink a glass of warm water before going to sleep. Warm water will help stave off night cramps, relieve pain, and helps to rid the body of unwanted toxins. This is because warm water is great for circulation. It will also keep you hydrated during the long hours of the night which in turn will help you have a good quality night's rest.

# Healthy Breakfast Ideas

The following are a few quick and simple healthy breakfast ideas to help kick start your morning.

## *Fasting Without Limited Calories*

This is usually done during the evening and into mid-morning the following day. If it does span a day there are non-fasting windows where a person can eat normally. See the non-fasting healthy ideas for normal eating day breakfast ideas.

## *Fasting With Limited Calories (100 to 130 Calories)*

The following recipes are 130 calories and under.

### Blueberry Mango Yogurt - 97 Calories

- 1 small mango chopped
- 1 oz blueberries (fresh or frozen)
- 4 tbsp non-fat plain Greek yogurt
- dash of ground cinnamon

Spoon the yogurt into a parfait glass or dessert bowl, add the chopped mango and blueberries. Add a dash of cinnamon for taste and to add a bit of sweetness.

## Egg White Mushroom Scramble - 93 Calories

- 3 tbsp fresh button mushrooms chopped
- 3 fresh egg whites
- 1 tsp coconut oil to cook with
- low-sodium salt and black pepper to taste

Heat the coconut oil in a skillet over medium heat. Add the egg whites and mushrooms stir into a scramble then serve hot.

## Cold Watermelon, Grapefruit, Kiwi, and Pomegranate Cup - 100 Calories

- 1 tbsp pomegranate seeds
- ½ small chopped kiwi fruit
- ½ small grapefruit
- ¼ cup iced, cubed fresh watermelon

Freeze the watermelon the night before. Add all the chopped fruit to a cereal or dessert bowl and enjoy a fresh fruit salad for breakfast.

## Almonds, Banana, and Honey - 129 Calories

- 1 small banana sliced
- 1 tbsp organic coconut flakes
- 1 tsp organic honey

Slice the banana and add it to a cereal or dessert bowl. Drizzle with organic honey, sprinkle over the coconut flakes and enjoy.

## Mixed Berry Coconut Smoothie - 121 Calories

- 3 tbsp blueberries
- 3 tbsp raspberries
- 3 tbsp blackberries
- 2 tsp shredded unsweetened coconut shreds
- ¼ cup unsweetened coconut water
- ½ cup still mineral water
- 1 tsp organic honey
- dash of cinnamon to taste

Add all the ingredients into a blender. Blend until the smoothie is thick and smooth. Add to a glass and drink or pack it in a container to take with you.

## *Healthy Breakfast Ideas for Normal Eating Days (500 Calories and Under)*

These easy breakfast recipes are filled with nutrients and are only 500 calories or less.

## Boiled Egg, Avocado, and Red Radish, Rocket Breakfast Salad - 471 Calories

- ½ avocado cubed
- ¼ cucumber sliced
- ¼ cup of rocket
- ¼ cup baby spinach leaves
- 3 large radishes sliced into rounds
- 2 hard-boiled eggs, halved

- 4 tbsp fat-free chunky cottage cheese
- low-sodium salt and black pepper to taste
- 1 slice wholewheat toast
- 1 tsp low-fat unsalted butter
- 1 tbsp balsamic vinegar

Add all the fresh ingredients to a salad bowl, toss, and drizzle with balsamic vinegar, add low-sodium salt and black pepper to taste. Halve the hard-boiled eggs and place them on top of the salad. Spread the whole wheat toast with the teaspoon of butter and serve with the salad.

## Spicy Mashed Sardines Mixed with Feta and Pickles on Whole Wheat Toast - 382 Calories

- 5 tbsp sardines, drained and mashed
- 2 slices of whole wheat toast
- 1 tbsp feta cheese
- 2 diced pickles
- 2 tsp butter
- dash of cayenne pepper to taste and add a zing

Mash the sardines with the feta and diced pickles add a dash of cayenne pepper for zing. Toast two slices of whole wheat bread and spread each one with the butter. Divide the sardines and spread onto each slice of toast to enjoy.

## Chocolate, Mixed Berry, Banana, Apricot, and Oats Breakfast Smoothie - 243 Calories

- 4 tbsp rolled oats
- 5 tbsp dried apricots
- 2 tbsp raspberries
- 2 tbsp blackberries
- ¼ cup chopped strawberries
- ½ small banana chopped
- 2 tsp organic honey
- ¼ unsweetened coconut water
- ¼ cup filtered water
- 2 tsp fresh chopped mint
- 1 tsp raw organic cocoa

Blend all the ingredients together until the smoothie is thick and smooth. Add to a glass and drink or pack it in a container to take with you.

## Tuna, Capers, Rocket, and Feta Omelet - 482 Calories

- 3 fresh eggs
- 4 tbsp canned tuna in water without added salt
- 2 tbsp feta cheese
- 4 tbsp chopped rocket
- 2 tbsp baby spinach leaves
- 1 tsp capers
- 1 slice whole wheat toast
- 1 tsp butter
- 1 tsp coconut oil cook with

- black pepper to taste

Scramble the eggs in a bowl. Heat the coconut oil in an omelet pan. Add the egg until it is almost completely cooked through. Add the tuna, feta, chopped rocket, baby spinach leaves, and capers to the one half of the egg mixture. Flip the free half over the ingredients to form an omelet fold. Cook on both sides for 1 to 2 minutes until the omelet is cooked through.

Toast the whole wheat bread and use the butter to spread it. Cut it into triangle halves and serve it with the hot omelet.

## Banana, Pomegranate Granola - 459 Calories

- 4 tbsp pomegranate seeds
- 1 large banana sliced
- 1 cup organic unsweetened granola
- 2 tsp organic honey
- 4 tbsp vanilla low-fat Greek yogurt
- 1 tbsp sunflower seeds
- 1 tbsp shredded unsweetened coconut

Place the granola in a cereal bowl. Top with the Greek yogurt and sliced banana. Drizzle the honey over the granola and banana. Top with pomegranate seeds, sunflower seeds, and shredded coconut.

# Healthy Lunch Ideas

Lunch is an important meal as it is the one that staves off the mid-morning hunger and gets you through the rest of the day. If you are going to eat a big meal, this would be a better time of the day to eat it. As you have to get through the next half of the day until supper you will be more likely to burn off most of the meal.

## *Fasting Without Limited Calories*

This is usually done during the evening and into mid-morning the following day. This means that your normal eating window would start at around 11 am. See the non-fasting healthy ideas for normal eating day lunch ideas. Try and cut down on the calories in order to help keep your system balanced. Instead of wolfing down a large amount of food because you have just come off a fast, drink a glass or two of water before eating. This will make you feel full and then go about preparing your meal.

## *Fasting With Limited Calories (200 to 250 Calories)*

The following lunches will go down well on fasting days with limited calories as they are all 250 calories and under.

## Beets, Ginger, Spring Onion With Grilled Hake - 127 Calories

- 1 grilled hake steak
- ¼ cup shredded raw beets
- 2 tbsp shredded fresh ginger root
- 3 spring onions chopped
- 1 tsp chili spice
- low-sodium salt and black pepper to taste

Preheat the grill. Prepare the hake steak with low-sodium salt, black pepper, and chili spice. Place in the grill and cook until the steak is almost done, about 10 to 15 minutes. Turn the steak halfway through cooking to cook evenly. Top with shredded ginger root and spring onion. Place the dish back into the grill for another 5 to 8 minutes. Remove from the grill, dish up onto a plate and top with fresh beets.

## Golden Chocolate Avocado Smoothie - 171 Calories

- ¼ chopped avocado
- ¼ small chopped banana
- 1 cup of filtered water
- ½ cup of ice cubes
- 1 tsp turmeric
- 1 tsp raw organic cocoa
- 1 tsp vanilla extract

Add all the ingredients into the blender. Blend until the smoothie is thick and smooth.

## Chicken and Avocado in a Kale Wrap - 223 Calories

- ¼ avocado sliced
- ¼ cup shredded grilled chicken breast
- 2 large kale leaves
- 1 tbsp smooth cottage cheese
- low-sodium salt and black pepper to taste

Mix the salt and pepper with the cottage cheese. Mix the shredded chicken and avocado into the cottage cheese mix. Wash and pat the kale leaves dry then stack them on top of each other. Add the shredded chicken, avocado, and cottage cheese into the middle of the top kale leaf. Fold the leaf into a wrap over the mixture and enjoy. You can make three small wraps if you prefer.

## Chicken Liver Stuffed Zucchini Boats - 198 Calories

- 1 large zucchini
- 4 tbsp cooked chicken livers
- 2 tbsp parmesan cheese
- ¼ cup mixed salad leaves
- 1 tsp pine nuts
- ¼ cherry tomatoes halved
- 1 tbsp feta cheese
- 2 tbsp pomegranate seeds
- 3 tsp balsamic vinegar
- low-sodium salt and black pepper to taste

Preheat the grill. Halve the zucchini cutting longways into two boats. Cut out a hollow (do not go right through the zucchini) in the middle of each boat. Put the cut-out zucchini flesh aside. Add the cooked chicken livers to the middle of the zucchini, dividing them evenly between the halves. Sprinkle parmesan over the top of the chicken livers, flavor with salt, and pepper. Place the zucchini boats into the grill for 8 to 10 minutes until cooked.

While the zucchini is cooking add the rest of the ingredients into a salad bowl, toss, and drizzle with balsamic vinegar. Add the extra zucchini cut out from the middle of the boat to the salad (chop into cubes). Flavor with salt and pepper to taste. When the zucchini boats are done serve with the salad.

## Eggplant Jalapeno and Prawn Pizza Slices— 219 Calories

- 1 large eggplant
- 2 tsp jalapeno peppers
- 6 cleaned, grilled king prawns
- 1 tbsp organic unsweetened tomato paste
- 1 tbsp shredded mozzarella cheese
- 1 tbsp parmesan cheese

Preheat the oven to 340°F. Peel the eggplant and slice long ways into slices (not too thin). Spread tomato paste on one side of each slice. Top the tomato paste with shredded mozzarella. Chop the prawns into bits and place them on top of the tomato paste along with the jalapeno peppers. Sprinkle a good coating of parmesan over each pizza slice. Place on a prepared baking tray and put into the oven to bake until cooked.

## Healthy Lunch Ideas for Normal Eating Days (500 Calories and Under)

### Tuna and Chunky Cottage Cheese Baked Potato with a Green Salad - 383 Calories

- 1 can tuna in water without salt drained
- 2 tbsp chunky fat-free plain cottage cheese
- 1 large Idaho baking potato
- ¼ cup mixed salad leaves
- ¼ cucumber diced
- ¼ green bell pepper diced
- 2 tbsp pumpkin seeds
- 2 tsp fresh basil
- 3 tsp organic balsamic vinegar
- low-sodium salt and black pepper to taste

Add salt and pepper to the cottage cheese, mix in the tuna. Bake the potato and scoop out the middle and mix with the tuna mixture. Add the tuna mixture to the middle of the baked potato. Toss the salad ingredients (salad leaves, cucumber, bell pepper, pumpkin seeds, and fresh basil). Add salt and pepper to taste, drizzle with balsamic vinegar and serve with the baked potato.

### Muscles, Lettuce, Capers, and Tomato Pita - 423 Calories

- 1 can of muscles, drained
- ¼ cup fresh shredded lettuce

- 1 whole wheat pita
- 1 tsp capers
- ½ large tomato diced
- 4 spring onions chopped
- ¼ cucumber diced
- 4 tsp smooth cottage cheese
- 1 tsp Dijon mustard
- ¼ tsp cayenne pepper

Mix together the cottage cheese, Dijon mustard, and cayenne pepper. Slice the top of the pita open and toast it until golden brown. In a bowl toss together the muscles, lettuce, capers, tomatoes, onions, and cucumber. Mix in the mayonnaise and Dijon mustard mix. Stuff the pita pocket with muscle mixture and enjoy it.

## Toasted Chicken and Hot English Mustard Mayo Sandwich - 464 Calories

- 2 slices of whole wheat bread
- ½ cup of shredded grilled chicken breast
- 1 tbsp low-fat mayonnaise
- 1 tsp hot English mustard
- 1 cup of oven chips
- 2 tsp unsalted butter

Cook the oven chips and spice with Cajun spice if desired. Mix together the low-fat mayonnaise and hot English mustard. Add the shredded grilled chicken to the mayonnaise and mustard mix. Use the unsalted butter to butter the bread. Place the chicken on one slice of the bread, cover with the other slice and grill the sandwich until it is toasted.

**Tuna, Prawn, Crab, and Lobster Salad - 429 Calories**

- 6 king prawns cleaned and grilled
- 4 tbsp fresh cooked crab meat
- 4 tbsp fresh cooked lobster meat
- 1 tsp capers
- 1 tsp jalapeno peppers
- 2 tsp sliced olives
- ¼ cup mixed salad leaves
- 2 tbsp feta
- ½ avocado diced
- 1 tbsp sesame seeds
- 3 tbsp low-fat mayonnaise
- 2 tsp Dijon mustard
- 1 tsp organic balsamic vinegar
- 1 tsp tomato ketchup
- 1 tsp organic honey

In a small mixing bowl mix together the low-fat mayonnaise, Dijon mustard, ketchup, honey, and balsamic vinegar. In a salad bowl, toss together the salad ingredients including the seafood. Drizzle with the mustard salad dressing and enjoy.

## Grilled Portobello Mushrooms with Feta Cheese and Avocado Bun - 500 Calories

- 1 large portobello mushroom
- 1 tbsp feta cheese
- 1 large avocado
- 1 cup tortilla chips
- 2 tsp sliced olives
- low-sodium salt and pepper to taste

Cut the stalk from the portobello mushroom and place it on a grilling dish with the stalk side up. Add some garlic flakes, low-sodium salt, and crumble feta cheese over the mushrooms. Place it on the grill and cook it until it starts to get soft and the feta has melted. Peel and cut the avocado in half longwise. Take out the pip, place the mushroom on the one half of the avocado. Cover the mushroom with the other half of the avocado making an avocado burger. Sever with 1 cup of tortilla chips and spice as desired.

## Healthy Dinner Ideas

Dinner should be a hearty meal, especially if you are going to be fasting the next day or through the nighttime into the next day. Try to eat earlier in the evening to avoid going to bed and a full stomach as this will be hard to digest and may give your problems sleeping.

## Fasting Without Limited Calories

Depending on your eating window this will probably be your second meal of the day during a fasting period. See the non-fasting healthy ideas for normal eating day dinner ideas. Once again try to control your portion sizes and gradually cut them down. Rather have a larger lunch than a larger dinner.

Try to eat before 7:30 pm in the evening.

## Fasting With Limited Calories (170 to 250 Calories)

The following are deliciously healthy dinner meals that offer optimum nutrition for under 250 calories.

### Ham and Cottage Cheese Chickpea Burger - 250 Calories

- 1 whole wheat burger bun
- 1 tbsp chopped cooked ham
- 2 tsp fat-free cottage cheese
- 1/4 cup mashed chickpeas
- 2 lettuce leaves
- ¼ tsp hot sauce

Drain and mash the chickpeas. Add the cottage cheese, hot sauce, and ham to the chickpea mixture. Pat the chickpea mixture into a burger patty shape. Grill for 8 to 10 minutes or until the chickpea patty has heated through. Halve the burger bun, place a lettuce leaf on each half. Put the chickpea patty on the bottom half, close the two halves and enjoy your burger.

**Grilled Tuna on One Potato Mash - 239 Calories**

- 1 Idaho potato, boiled, and mashed
- 1 grilled tuna steak
- 1 cup of baby spinach leaves
- 1 tsp pine nuts
- 1 tbsp feta cheese
- 1 tsp sunflower seeds
- 1 tsp raw chopped cashew nuts
- 2 tsp organic balsamic vinegar

Grill the tuna, seasoned with low-sodium salt and black pepper to taste. Boil and mash the Idaho potato. Toss the spinach leaves, pine nuts, sunflower seeds, cashews and feta in a salad bowl then drizzle with balsamic vinegar. Serve the tuna on top of the mash with the green salad on the side.

**Vegetable and 3 Cheese Tart - 215 Calories per serving**

- ½ eggplant
- 3 courgettes
- ½ red bell pepper
- ½ cup baby spinach leaves
- 2 tbsp olive slices
- 1 tbsp jalapeno peppers
- 1 roll of puff pastry
- 4 tbsp feta cheese

- 4 tbsp fat-free cottage cheese
- 2 tbsp parmesan cheese

This makes three servings.

Preheat the oven to 300°F. Prepare a baking tray with cooking spray. Roll out the filo pastry and place it in a pie shape at the bottom of the baking tray. Place the pastry into the oven until it starts to get brown. Cook the vegetables in a skillet with coconut oil over medium heat. When cooked, mix in the cream cheese and place them in the pie crust. Mix in olive slices and crumble feta over the vegetable mix. Sprinkle with parmesan cheese and place the pie back in the oven for another 8 to 10 minutes until the cheese has melted in. Remove from the oven and serve.

## Asparagus, Green Bean, and Poached Egg Salad - 218 Calories

- 5 fresh grilled asparagus spears
- 1 cup grilled green beans
- 2 poached egg
- ½ cup baby spinach leaves
- ¼ cup rocket
- 4 tsp Dijon mustard

Lay a bed of baby spinach leaves mixed with rocket leaves. Place the grilled asparagus and beans onto the mixed leaves. Place the warm poached egg on the top, drizzle with Dijon mustard and enjoy.

## Grilled Turkey Breast with Boiled Garlic and Ginger Butter Baby Potatoes - 250 Calories

- 4 washed and boiled baby potatoes
- ½ grilled turkey breast cut into slices
- 1 tsp grated fresh ginger root
- 1 tsp organic crushed garlic
- 3 tsp unsalted butter
- low-sodium salt and black pepper to taste

Place the hot grilled and sliced turkey breast on a plate with the boiled baby potatoes. In a pot melt the butter with the grated ginger root and garlic. When the butter is cooked, pour the mixture over the baby potatoes and serve. You can add some mixed salad leaves if you wish.

## *Dinner Ideas for Normal Eating Days (500 Calories and Under)*

The following dinner ideas are quick and easy to make, are under 500 calories and high in healthy nutrition.

## Bison Burger with Cajun Oven Baked Potato Wedges and Sour Cream - 500 Calories

- 1 bison burger patty
- 1 whole wheat bun
- 1 tbsp Dijon mustard
- 1 large pickle, thinly sliced

- 1 large washed lettuce leaf
- 1 slice of a large tomato
- 1 cup of oven-baked potato wedges
- 1 tsp Cajun spice
- 3 tbsp low-fat sour cream
- 1 tsp finely chopped fresh dill

Halve the burger bun and spread each half with Dijon mustard. Grill the bison burger patty and before stacking it on the bottom of the halved burger bun. Top the patty with a lettuce leaf, tomato slice, sliced pickle. In a bowl, mix together the sour cream and dill. Bake the potato wedges according to the pack, spice with Cajun spice and drizzle with the sour cream and fresh chive sauce.

## Surf and Turf with a Baked Potato and Sour Cream - 500 Calories

- 1 prime cut steak - grilled and spiced to your liking
- 1 large baking potato, baked until soft
- 6 large grilled prawns
- 1 tsp garlic butter
- 1 tsp unsalted butter
- 1 tbsp sour cream
- 1 cup cooked green beans

Cook the steak and baking potato to your liking. Grill the prawns and heat the garlic butter when the prawns are nearly cooked. Cook the green beans to your liking and serve them onto a dinner plate. Add the steak, prawns, and baked potatoes. Pour the heated garlic butter over the prawns. Add unsalted butter, sour cream, salt, and pepper to the baked potato and serve while nice and hot.

**Quick Black Bean Chili - 343 Calories**

- ¼ cup of cooked brown rice
- ½ white onion chopped
- 2 large fresh tomatoes chopped
- 1 can black beans
- 2 tsp crushed garlic
- 1 tbsp of chili powder (strength to your taste)
- 2 tbsp of organic honey
- 2 tbsp jalapeno peppers
- 2 tbsp organic balsamic vinegar
- 2 tsp paprika
- 2 tbsp sour cream
- 4 tbsp of feta
- ½ thinly sliced avocado
- 8 sprigs of fresh mint
- ¼ cup of warm water

This recipe makes 4 servings.

Cook the rice when the chili has fifteen minutes of cooking time left. In a large pot bring the warm water to boil, add the onion, black beans, crushed garlic, chili powder, honey, balsamic vinegar, and paprika. Allow the chili to cook for 1 hour 30 minutes or until the beans are soft. Serve with a dollop of sour cream, crumbled feta, avocado, and some fresh mint.

## Avocado, Bacon, Rocket, and Feta Tortilla Pizza - 342 Calories

- 1 whole wheat tortilla
- ¼ avocado thinly sliced
- ¼ cup crisped bacon pieces
- 4 tbsp rocket
- 2 tbsp feta
- 4 tbsp shredded mozzarella
- 2 tsp organic tomato paste
- low-sodium salt and black pepper to taste

Preheat the oven to 340°F. Spread the tortilla with tomato paste, top with mozzarella, avocado, bacon, rocket, and crumble the feta cheese over the top. Place it in the oven and cook until all the ingredients are cooked, and the tortilla is golden brown.

## Spicy Mince Meat Pancakes - 370 Calories

- Make a pancake mixture (2 eggs, ¼ cup flour, ¼ cup reduced-fat milk)
- 1 cup mince
- 5 basil leaves
- 1 tsp dried oregano
- 1 tsp chili powder
- 1 tsp jalapeno peppers
- 1 tsp capers
- ¼ cup mixed salad leaves
- ¼ cucumber chopped
- 1 celery stalk chopped

- 1 tsp balsamic vinegar

Make two pancakes. Cook the mince with the herbs and spices. Dish the mince out evenly into the middle of each pancake. Add jalapeno peppers and capers to each pancake and serve. Toss the salad greens together (salad leaves, cucumber, and celery) then drizzle balsamic vinegar over them. Serve the pancakes with the green salad on the side.

## Healthy Smoothies

These smoothies can be used to replace breakfast or lunch. They can also be used as a snack.

Smoothies are fun to make and you can experiment with different fruit, nut, and vegetable blends. Add different types of nut milk, nut creams, yogurt, and so on. They are always tastier when you add seeds.

Keep the ingredients healthy and within snack or meal calorie requirements. They are a great way to get all your nutrition requirements in for the day. They can also be taken as an on the go meal or snack.

Smoothies may only be drunk during normal eating periods or windows. As they are a snack that contains carbs they cannot be drunk during the fasting periods.

They are easy to make as you put all the ingredients into a blender, then blend until smooth and thick. Leftover smoothie mixture can be kept in an airtight container in the refrigerator for up to two days.

Smoothies with added protein powder are a great way to aid muscle recovery after a tough workout, long run, bike ride, etc. They can also give you that added boost of energy if you are feeling tired and run down.

### *Smoothie Ingredients*

Smoothies can contain any fruit, berry, nut, seed, protein whey powder, yogurt, etc.

Fruit and berries can be either frozen or fresh. Avoid canned fruit or berries and check that the products do not have any added sugar, flavors, or colorants.

Here are a few examples of the most popular smoothie ingredients:

**Berries**

- Raspberries
- Blackberries
- Blueberries
- Strawberries

**Fruit**

- Banana (they are great for thickening and sweetening a smoothie)
- Avocado

- Pear
- Plum
- Peach
- Apple
- Pineapple
- Melon (yellow)
- Papaya
- Watermelon
- Grapes
- Pomegranate seeds
- Kiwi
- Mango
- Coconut

## Nuts

- Cashews
- Macadamia
- Walnuts
- Almonds
- Pecan
- Pistachios
- Brazil nuts

## Seeds

- Chia
- Sunflower
- Pinenut
- Pumpkin

- Sesame
- Fennel

## Vegetables

- Kale
- Spinach
- Cabbage
- Broccoli
- Tomato
- Celery
- Carrot
- Raddish
- Horseradish
- Cucumber
- Spring onion
- Artichoke
- Garlic
- Rocket
- Capers

## Herbs

- Mint
- Basil
- Oregano
- Parsley
- Ginger
- Rosemary
- Cardamom

- Mustard seeds
- Chives

## Spices

- Turmeric
- Paprika
- Cayenne pepper
- Ground cinnamon
- Allspice
- Chili powder
- Chili seeds
- Ground ginger
- Garlic powder
- Cumin
- Dill
- Low sodium salt
- Black pepper
- White pepper
- Worcestershire sauce
- Soy sauce
- Hot sauce
- Tomato ketchup
- Mustard

## Liquids

- Filtered water
- Ice cubes
- Almond milk

- Hemp milk
- Rice milk
- Oat milk
- Coconut milk
- Coconut cream
- Coconut water
- Low-fat milk
- Cream
- Fruit juice
- Vegetable juice

## Other

- Vanilla essence
- Pure vanilla
- Organic Balsamic vinegar
- Curry powder
- Vegetable oil
- Protein whey powder (all flavors)
- Plain low-fat Greek yogurt
- Low-fat cream cheese
- Fat-free cottage cheese
- Flavored low-fat yogurt
- Sugar-free ice cream (all flavors)
- Raw organic cocoa powder
- Dark chocolate chips
- Dark chocolate blocks
- Organic honey

- Desiccated coconut
- Coconut flakes
- Fresh chilis

*Smoothie Ideas*

These are tasty smoothies that are full of good nutrition, taste great and 350 calories or under.

## Avocado, Banana, Chocolate, and Ginger Smoothie - 312 Calories

- ½ banana
- ½ avocado
- 1 tbsp grated fresh ginger root
- 1 tsp sunflower seeds
- 1 tsp chia seeds
- 1 tsp vanilla extract
- ¼ cup unsweetened almond milk
- ¼ cup of filtered water

## Peach, Blueberry Cheesecake Smoothie - 350 Calories

- ½ banana
- 1 peach
- ½ cup blueberries
- 1 tbsp sesame seeds
- 1 tbsp organic honey
- ½ cup low-fat milk

- ¼ cup of ice cubes
- ¼ cup sugar-free vanilla ice cream

## The Green and Gold Smoothie - 124 Calories

- ½ banana
- ¼ cup kale
- ¼ cup baby spinach leaves
- ¼ cucumber
- ½ green bell pepper
- 1 tsp fresh dill
- 2 tsp turmeric
- ½ cup of filtered water
- ¼ cup unsweetened coconut water
- low-sodium salt and black pepper to taste

## Berry, Nut, and Seed Coconut Cream Smoothie with a Zing - 319 Calories

- ¼ cup blackberries
- ¼ cup blueberries
- ¼ cup raspberries
- ¼ cup pomegranate seeds
- 1 tsp sunflower seeds
- 1 tsp fennel seeds
- 1 tsp sesame seeds
- 3 tsp raw cashew nuts
- 2 tsp pecan nuts
- 2 tbsp unsweetened shredded coconut
- 4 tbsp unsweetened coconut cream

- ¼ cup unsweetened almond milk
- ¼ cup of filtered water
- 3 tsp organic honey
- dash of cayenne pepper

## Tomato Beet Vegetable Cocktail Smoothie - 154 Calories

- 1 carrot
- 2 celery stalks
- 2 medium tomatoes
- ¼ cup baby spinach leaves
- ½ green bell pepper
- ¼ cucumber
- ¼ cup grated fresh beets
- 3 tsp fresh basil
- ½ cup of filtered water
- ¼ cup fresh orange juice
- low-sodium salt and ground black pepper to taste

## Tropical Coconut Cream and Ginger Smoothie - 350 Calories

- ½ cup of pineapple
- ½ banana
- ½ mango
- 1 kiwifruit
- ¼ papaya
- 1 tbsp unsweetened shredded coconut
- 1 tbsp grated ginger root
- 1 tsp ground cinnamon

- 2 tsp organic honey
- ¼ cup fresh orange juice
- ¼ cup fresh lime juice

# Beverages During Fasting Periods

There are some beverages you can drink during fasting periods and some you must avoid. There are also substances that must not be added to any beverages during fast and substances that can be added.

Here are some ideas on what you should and should not be drinking during fasting periods.

## *Water*

Water should be drunk continuously during the day even when you are not fasting.

Water is always best drunk as natural, filtered, or spring water that can be either carbonated or still.

### You May Add

- Lemon
- Lime
- Cucumber slices
- The water can be carbonated

## You May Not Add

- Artificial sweeteners
- Colorants
- Artificial flavors
- Fruit
- Berries

## *Tea*

There are a few teas that should be avoided and those that can be consumed. It is best to drink the tea black with a bit of cold water if it needs to be cooled down.

## You May Drink the Following Tea

- Oolong tea
- Black tea
- Normal tea
- Green tea
- Cinnamon tea
- Peppermint tea
- Spearmint tea

## You May Add

- Stevia
- Cinnamon
- Nutmeg
- Lemon juice

**You May Not Add**

- Artificial sweeteners
- Milk
- Cream
- Artificial flavors
- Fruit
- Herbs
- Spices

## Coffee

Black coffee helps to keep you alert and awake. It also can aid in weight loss.

**You May Add**

- Stevia
- Cinnamon
- Nutmeg
- Lemon juice

**You May Not Add**

- Artificial sweeteners
- Milk
- Cream
- Artificial flavors
- Herbs
- Spices

# Concerns During Fasting

One of the major causes of people giving up fasting is because they get headaches, feel nauseous, or cannot stave off hunger.

Here are a few tips to help get you through a few concerns.

## *Constipation*

Constipation does happen during fasting, especially when you first start out.

Try these tips:

- Increase your fiber content during your eating windows.
- Drink carbonated water.
- Use fennel seeds with your smoothies or sprinkle them over your food.
- Drink hot coffee.
- Drink black or green tea.

## *Dizziness*

You may feel a bit dizzy or like you have vertigo during the fasting periods. You may even feel light-headed every time you stand up or get a blood rush to the head. This is usually caused by dehydration.

Try these tips:

- Increase your fluid intake.
- Drink mint in your water during the eating windows.
- Take liver salts during the eating window.
- Cut down on coffee and tea intake for a while.

## *Fatigue or Lethargy*

You will feel a bit fatigued or lethargic during fasting periods. You could also be lacking some vital nutrients. Increase your nutrient intake during non-fasting periods.

Try these tips:

- Increase your fluid intake.
- Eat high energy foods during your eating window and at least an hour before your fasting period is about to start.
- Splash cold water on your face.
- Do some light exercise.
- Take supplements during your eating window.

## *Headaches*

Headaches are another common occurrence during fasting. Your body goes through a period of withdrawal and is not used to being starved of food.

Try these tips:

- Drink more water.

- Drink mineral water during your non-fasting periods.

### Muscle Cramps or Spasms

Fasting also means cutting down salt and some minerals. This can cause muscle cramps and muscle spasms.

Try these tips:

- Take Epsom salts twice a week during your eating windows.
- Increase your magnesium intake during your eating windows.

### Nausea

You may experience nausea if hunger sets in or you may experience migraine symptoms.

Try these tips:

- Drink peppermint tea.
- Drink liver salts during your eating window.

### Hunger

The most common concern or complaint is feeling hungry. There is a lot you can do to stop you from feeling hungry and to relieve the hunger pangs.

Try these tips:

- Increase your fiber content during your eating windows.
- Eat more slow-release carbs at least an hour before the fasting period begins.
- Drink carbonated water.
- Drink green tea.
- Drink coffee.
- Add cinnamon to your coffee or tea.
- Distract yourself by keeping busy with a hobby.
- Get some light exercise in or go for a long walk.
- Meditate.
- Go visit a friend.

### *Sleeping Problems*

If you are fasting during the night you would have probably started fasting around 7:30 pm. Move that up to at least 9 pm and have a light snack and cup of chamomile tea before bed.

Read a book and turn off all electronics that may be disturbing your sleeping pattern. Make sure your room is cool, even in winter your room needs to be cool in order to maintain a quality sleep pattern.

Keep a fresh bottle of water next to your bed in case you get thirsty during the night so you do not have to get up and go pour one.

Learn sleep meditation to relax your body and help you drift off to sleep.

# Chapter 8: Maintaining Your Weight

Intermittent fasting should become a way of life and once you have started it, you should try to do it at least twice a month or every other month. After all, you are going to want to maintain your weight once you have reached your goal.

## After Diet Natural Appetite Control

Once you have reached your goal weight, you will need to keep a maintenance diet plan. Try to keep your calories under control; at first it may seem like hard work, but it eventually becomes second nature.

Fasting should be on your list of things to do every now and then, or at least once a month. At first, when you start fasting, it is going to be hard, but persevere, drink water as it will help to keep you energized as well as awake.

If you keep fasting, you will soon start to feel the benefits of intermittent fasting. Your body will feel lighter, you will begin to be able to identify the signs of actual hunger. Once your body becomes used to fasting, you will be able to navigate fasting times without too much hunger. Eat food that keeps you fuller for longer and keep well hydrated, you will start to have more energy and feel healthier.

A natural way to contain hunger is to drink water before meals as it will fill you up and you will not eat too much. Try to cut back on snacks and only eat when you feel real hunger pangs. Instead of eating unhealthy snacks or sweets rather eat a piece of fruit or a handful of nuts.

Eat good carbs and whole foods instead of processed or sugary foods. For more energy, eat foods such as a banana's, avocado's, or a whole-wheat sandwich. These foods will keep you fuller for that much longer. Don't forget to hydrate, as water does wonders for the body, the skin, and even your hair. Listen to your body. It will let you know what it needs and the more you fast, the more in tune you will become with it.

## Lowered Levels of Inflammation in the Body

The body is not really designed to have three large meals a day and then snacks in between. If we have learned anything from history, it is that our ancestors would go out foraging for food. There were times when food was in abundance and then times when it was not. So, they would either feast or go hungry for days at a time occasionally.

As they did not have the fancy tools or cooling equipment as we are fortunate to have these days, they could not store their food either. We do not only need sleep to keep us alert and give us downtime, we need it so our body can perform vital housekeeping functions. These housekeeping functions are made more difficult when we abuse our systems with bad food or too much food.

There have been studies that showed intermittent fasting caused an anti-inflammatory response in the body after fasting for certain periods of time. These anti-inflammatory responses include the following (Papconstantinou, 2019):

- Increase cellular immune response.
- Improve gut microbiota composition.
- Reduce the risk of insulin resistance.

It also reduces the risk of diabetes, rheumatoid arthritis, and Alzheimer's as it keeps them at bay by producing a chemical compound called β-hydroxybutyrate. This chemical compound is used by the cells to produce energy when the body hits a low blood sugar. It also helps the brain function better as well as the body's nervous system. Mostly it seems to keep the immune system in check, so it does not cause diseases as previously mentioned.

Inflammation is measured by cytokines, C-reactive protein markers which intermittent fasting helps to reduce.

## Decreased Insulin Levels and Insulin Resistance

Studies have shown that fasting can significantly reduce body weight by up to 8% which is a start to getting insulin levels under control. The same studies showed that people who did alternate day fasting reduced their insulin levels by up to 52% and improved their insulin resistance by up to 53% (Arguin, Dionne, Sénéchal, Bouchard, Carpentier, Ardilouze, et al., 2012).

Although studies still continue and more research is needed before fasting will be clinically recommended, people who have followed an intermittent fasting diet have shown great results for a reduction in insulin levels and insulin resistance.

## Clean Food for a Clean Mindset

Clean eating is a concept whereby a person makes themselves aware of where the food came from and how it got to their plate. In other words, eating foods that are not processed, and contain no GMOs or pesticides. Food not only has to be cooked in cleaner, more natural ways, but it has to have been handled that way before it was bought too.

Making the more natural and healthy choice when choosing your foods means cutting out boxed, packaged, processed, bagged, or artificially colored and flavored foods. Instead of going for the can of fruit choose the organic fresh fruit. But people who have followed an intermittent fasting diet have shown great results for reduction in insulin levels and insulin resistance.

These foods are called whole foods and include fresh foods, whole grains, unrefined sugars, less dairy, and lower salt. All of which is a lot healthier, reduces the risk of disease, and improves a person's overall health. After a person becomes familiar with and used to fasting, they will want to make healthier choices as they start to feel cleaner on the inside.

At first, you may think it is quite the mission to make these choices but if you persevere and take the extra minute to read the back of a can or package you will notice all the added ingredients. Most of which you probably cannot even pronounce, and they are not natural. You are making the effort to become healthier, lose weight, and feel better so go the extra mile and make those better food choices.

Once you have tasted the difference in whole foods over-processed, refined, and artificially grown, flavored, or colored you will naturally avoid them. Eating clean reprograms both your mind and body to want cleaner foods.

# Chapter 9: Intermittent Fasting Foods

It is very, very important to hydrate while intermittent fasting as the body will process the sugar that is stored in the liver (glycogen) to burn as an energy source. When it burns glycogen, the body also loses a large volume of fluid which needs to be replenished.

Water is the best hydration for the body, and a person should drink at least the recommended daily dose of it, more if you are doing a lot of exercise.

Some of the foods and beverages to eat or drink when fasting should include:

- Unsweetened tea and coffee must be drunk without any flavoring or powdered milk substitutes.
- Water is the best beverage to drink as long as it is plain water with no flavoring. You can infuse the water with mint but cannot add anything to sweeten it.
- You will need carbohydrates to sustain you through the fasting periods so during the eating window try to eat whole grains.
- Potatoes constitute another significant source of food for the body and most white potatoes are easily digested by the body. They also promote good gut bacteria to help your digestion.

- Chickpeas are a very versatile food and can be eaten as a roasted snack or as hummus.
- Fruit, and vegetables (or a mixture of both) smoothies made with nut milk fill the body with needed nutrients and can also take away sweet cravings. They are filling and as long as you stick to healthy choices you can experiment with the flavors.
- Berries are a great snack and are so healthy, they are packed full of goodness. Try blueberries, raspberries, and blackberries. They are also filled with antioxidants and are another way of quelling sweet cravings.
- Nuts, eaten in moderation, are a great snack; they also complement many dishes. They aid the body in eliminating fat; they can also reduce the risk of type 2 diabetes and may increase longevity.
- Supplements are something to consider as you may not be consuming enough nutrients.
- Dairy products that are fortified with vitamin D as this is the one vitamin that most people tend to lack. You can get vitamin D by exposing your skin to at least 15 minutes in the sun a day. But there are places in the world where that is just not possible for long periods of the year. So look for healthy products that possess an adequate amount of vitamin D, which a lot of fortified milk products have.

# Intermittent Fasting Foods to Control Blood Sugar Levels

To control insulin levels during intermittent fasting, a person should include the following foods into their daily diet and eating windows:

- Fatty fish such as herring, salmon, sardines, mackerel, and anchovies contain a good quantity of Omega 3 fats. Fatty fish may lower a person's risk of heart disease as well as being good for blood sugar levels. It is also good for brain power as well as cuts down inflammation markers in the body.
- Eggs, not only help to reduce insulin levels but they are also one of the best foods to eat to keep a person fuller for longer. They are also good for reducing the risk of heart disease; it feeds the muscles, improves insulin resistance, and decreases inflammation markers.
- Greek yogurt is another food that helps to reduce blood sugar levels. It is also a very versatile food that can be used to replace mayonnaise. It can be used to thicken smoothies, replace ice cream, eaten as a dish on its own, or enjoyed as a dessert topped with berries.
- Strawberries are at the top of the list when it comes to nutritious fruits. They are very high in antioxidants, especially the one that gives them their color called anthocyanin. Anthocyanin may reduce the risk of heart

disease, reduce cholesterol, and can lower blood sugar after a meal.

- Nuts contain fiber. They also have low digestible carbs which make them a great low-carb option. There are some nuts though that are a bit more carbs than others. But a person should include cashews, Brazil nuts, hazelnuts, almonds, pistachio, walnuts, and pecans.

- Turmeric is something that a person should try to incorporate into their meal even if they do not need to control blood sugar. It has cancer-fighting properties as well as reduces the risk of heart disease besides being a natural component for controlling insulin levels.

- Seeds such as flax seeds have great fiber in them to help reduce insulin levels. Chia seeds are another great seed source filled with fiber and compounds that not only reduce insulin but also the risk of heart disease and cancer.

- Leafy green vegetables like spinach, lettuce, and kale help to control insulin levels while also reducing the risk of heart disease. They are also packed with vitamins and nutrients that the body needs, especially during fasting.

- Garlic is not just to add flavor to a meal it has many great health properties to it as well. These include helping to control insulin levels, fighting cancer, and reducing the risk of heart disease.

- Cinnamon should somehow be inserted into a person's daily diet as it has so much to offer. One benefit, in particular, is that it helps to control insulin levels after meals.

- Squash is a food that does not get all the mention it should. All kinds of squash such as butternut, pumpkin, zucchini, and various summer squashes to help not only control insulin levels but obesity too.
- Broccoli is another food that a lot of people really do not like. They prefer to go for cauliflower. While cauliflower has its benefits, broccoli is an easily digestible carb that contains vitamins C along with other much-needed nutrients and vitamins.

## Detox Food for Energy and Vitality

Some foods can help in detoxing the system. Then there are those foods a person should avoid if trying to detox.

Foods to avoid include:

- Dairy products are acidic which can slow down the detoxification process as these products can lead to the cells not functioning as they should.
- Alcohol should be avoided at all costs as it is toxic and affects the liver. Alcohol reduces levels of magnesium and zinc which are products needed for detoxification.
- Meat does not get digested very fast and promotes the breeding of bacteria in the gut. This bacteria is not the good kind either. Meat tends to clog up the system as it is

hard for the body to digest so it takes longer, thus slowing down the digestion.

- Caffeine is also harmful as it has been known to increase toxicity in the body.
- Salt is also not too good for the body and can raise a person's blood pressure. High blood pressure causes a lot of damage and increases the risk of a stroke. It is not good for detoxing either as it slows down normal cell function.
- Sugar should be avoided, especially processed sugar. Even brown sugar that is not organic has been processed. It also conflicts with the good bacteria in a person's gut which can be detrimental for detoxing. While sugar may give a person an instant rush of energy, it burns off really quickly which could leave you feeling drained afterward. It is also quite addictive as your body comes to crave the sugar rush.
- Avoid packaged foods or foods with artificial colors or flavors. Foods that contain a lot of salt or saturated fats must also be avoided.

Food to eat to encourage detox and boost your energy levels includes:

- Vegetables; if you can try to find organic vegetables and choose fresh rather than frozen.
- Berries are high in antioxidants. Fresh berries are always the better choice. Although frozen berries are just as good if sugar-free and with little to no preservatives.

- Whole grains are high in fiber which promotes gut health to aid digestion and keeps you feeling full.
- Most fruit is a great source of natural sugar. They not only aid in detoxing but also help to stave off sweet cravings. They are also full of vital vitamins and nutrients.
- Nuts and seeds are a great source of protein help to improve detoxing. They also contain many healthy nutrients. They also contain fat-soluble vitamins vital for feeding the brain.

## Anti-Aging Foods

One of the first places to show an indication of a problem within the human body is the skin. It is after all the largest organ of the body. A person can use all the topical lotions as well as potions but there is only so much they can do. The skin needs to heal and be rejuvenated from within the body through feeding it correctly.

One of the best ways to reduce fine lines, smooth out wrinkles, or eliminate those dark spots or lines is through eating correctly. A bright healthy glowing skin comes from within not from some potion or magical base cover you have applied to it.

To help encourage healthy skin and slow down the signs of aging your diet should include the following foods:

- Blueberries are supercharged foods that contain a good number of vitamins A and C. They also contain anthocyanin which is an antioxidant with age-defying properties. Blueberries are also a great way to sweeten plain yogurt or smoothies.

- Avocado contains some nutrients that have been known to slow down the effects of aging. These nutrients are potassium, vitamin K, vitamin C, Vitamin A, and B vitamins. They also contain helpful carotenoids that aid in stopping the harmful effects of the sun which in turn may help fight against skin cancer.

- Papaya is a superfood that contains a high content of minerals, vitamins, and antioxidants to improve the skin's appearance. Papaya may just be the superfood required to smooth out those fine lines or wrinkles and improve the skin's elasticity. It is also a rich source of vitamins E, vitamin K, vitamin A, vitamin C, potassium, calcium, magnesium, and B vitamins. It is one of the foods you should be trying to eat at least once or twice a week.

- Nuts and seeds make the list again as some nuts, like walnuts, contain Omega-3 fatty acids. Omega-3 has been known to help protect the skin against the harmful rays of the sun, create a natural glow, and help to strengthen the skin membranes.

- Pomegranate is another superfood that most people are unaware of but has been used in alternative medicines for centuries. They contain punicalagin which helps in the slowing down of the skin aging process as it protects collagen.

- Red bell peppers contain lots of vitamin C. Vitamin C is essential for the production of collagen. They also contain carotenoids which are well-known antioxidants.
- Leafy green vegetables, broccoli, and sweet potatoes are also vegetables that help to maintain the skin as they contain lots of vitamins and nutrients. These vitamins and nutrients are particularly helpful in protecting the skin from the harmful damage of the sun.

# Chapter 10: Changing Your Habits and Your Mindset to Change Your Body

The best way to get rid of old habits is to change your mindset.

## Take Control of Your Habits

Bad habits get ingrained into your subconscious as they are repeated day in and day out. Biting your nails, sucking your thumb, eating three large meals a day, and so on. Habits are created by routine patterns over a period of time. These habits are started by our parents growing up, by nerves, anxiety, or as a way of support. Breaking them does not happen in a day and will take time. Some habits you do not even know you are doing as they have become a reflex. This includes the way you eat, cook, and even shop.

Habits, no matter what they are, can be broken. You just need to want to break the habit, have the strength to push through breaking the habit, and believe that you can.

### Breaking Bad Habits

Instead of trying to break them, replace them with healthier ones.

Here are some tips on how to take control of your habits in order to change them.

## The Triggers

Become aware of your triggers. Once you are aware of why you do what you do, you can find a way around them. Habits are a person's little comfort devices and as such are really easy to fall back into. In order to change them, we need to develop new comforts and at midlife, it becomes quite a challenge to do.

One way to retrain the response to a trigger would be to have a countermeasure in place. For example, if you find yourself reaching for dessert after supper, stop and ask yourself why you are having the dessert. Are you still hungry? If so, go get something with less sugar and calories in, or reach for fruit instead.

If you are really wanting something sweet, have a glass of infused water and think about what healthy snacks you could eat instead. Grapes are a healthier alternative to sweets, chocolates, or carbonated drinks.

Don't think, "I must eat something healthy." Rather think, "I would much prefer something healthy to eat."

When you go shopping, don't think, "I must prefer to take this product." Reach for the healthier alternative and think "Ah! This is my new favorite brand."

## Dealing with Triggers

Most people are aware of their triggers on some level. The best solution would be to avoid situations that trigger bad habits. The thing is, in real life you are always going to come across a trigger or two somewhere. It is like trying to avoid a person you do not like, unless you are going to change continents, even then that is no guarantee.

If you cannot avoid them, learn how to deal with them. As per the section above, have a coping mechanism you can fall back on other than the bad habit. If you find you are unable to resist hotdogs, when you pass a hotdog vendor carry a nutritious snack with you. A few squares of dark chocolate could do the trick or a handful of berries or nuts. Take it out and eat it as you pass by or dial a friend to occupy your mind while you walk past.

Find a mantra that best suits you and talk yourself through it when you find yourself in a situation that triggers a habit. You are trying to combat the signs of aging, not just on the outside but on the inside. To do that you have to break the bad eating habits and that includes the way you cook, the groceries you buy, and eating out habits. Most decent restaurants and even fast-food places are trying to offer healthy menu choices. Think of trying something new on the menu for a new and improved you!

**Switching the Bad for the Good**

In theory, it sounds quite easy to do but in reality, it is really hard. You have spent most of your life eating the way you do, shopping the way you do, and so on. By now your life works on autopilot as you go through your habitual daily routine. Now you are trying to slowly change your entire lifestyle and undo all those years of mental wiring.

It is going to take strength, commitment, and perseverance. But the end results of intermittent fasting and opting for a healthier lifestyle really do justify the means. One of the best ways to start is to think of it as switching out this product for a new product. Kind of like switching out your laundry detergents to try a new brand. Don't think of it as breaking bad habits or a diet. Rather think of your new lifestyle as trying something new.

## Change Your Mindset

You have had a certain mindset for years and now you are changing it. Retraining your brain, setting new routines, and developing new comfort zones. The human psyche is complex, and humans really are their own worst enemies. Believe it or not, you are going to come up against resistance to all your changes. Even the smallest of changes may have some form of resistance. The hardest part is it is not resistance from a moody teenager or partner. The resistance to change will come from within you!

You can start to change your mindset by trying some of the following methods:

### Have a Clear Vision

One thing on your side, when you reach midlife, is that your taste changes. Usually, at midlife, a person starts to find that foods that once agreed with them no longer do. While other foods may become more appealing, your tastes can actually change and food may not taste the same. Now is the best time to embrace new eating habits. You have the perfect excuse to use against your inner rebel.

If eating meat has started to cause indigestion, try substituting it with a plant-based alternative. Chickpeas make a great, tasty, meat alternative. If you love bacon, you don't have to give it up entirely; once again try a plant alternative, like eggplant. Find the foods that best suit you and your new tastes, don't be afraid to try something new. This is a new phase of your life cycle. Not only are you turning over a new leaf, but you are getting to know this new you.

Parents will have gone through the different phases in their kid's life and as they grew you had to grow with them. You adapted and evolved around the different stages. This is a lot like that, only now you have reached a new phase of your life. To enjoy your golden years in optimum health, change is necessary. Even those that have led a relatively healthy lifestyle, trained every day, and conquered mountains, will have to adapt at this point in their life.

Your body is changing from the inside, and what worked for you before menopause will most likely no longer work for you now. You can't let it defeat you or get you down, you need to embrace it and set your vision as to where you go from here. Make a list of the most significant changes you feel you need to address. Include what you would like to change and note any health issues that you feel you need to address.

## Midlife Vision Board

Vision boards are a lot of fun and are really trending these days. They give you something to aspire to and as you notice changes during your lifestyle change it serves as a great visualization tool. There is nothing more motivating than actually seeing the changes and how much you have transformed from point A to where you currently are.

## Chart Your Progress

Set a date for once a week, bi-weekly, or monthly where you take note of your changes. Weigh yourself, measure yourself, take note of much further you can walk now, and so on. Document how you feel. Are you sleeping better? Do you feel like you have more energy now?

List all the changes you made for the time period, how you adapted to them, and any new changes or modifications you think you need.

Make sure to write down the times you slipped up, anything you had a hard time with and the things that just did not meet your needs. It may seem like hard work, but you will be amazed how encouraging it is when you lay it all out. It also gives you a baseline from which to work from and a way to make adjustments.

### Set Obtainable Goals

One of the worst things you can do is set your targets or goals too high. Keep a clear vision in mind of what your overall target is. Then set weekly or rather monthly targets to strive for.

Make weekly goals about small adjustments to your lifestyle, like changing dairy products for nut milk. Make your monthly targets about losing weight or rather centimeters and your fitness levels.

Breaking down your lifestyle goals into smaller obtainable and doable chunks makes achieving your overall goal more realistic. Having small goals is similar to breaking down a project into milestones. You know where the project is going and how it should end up and the steps to take to get there.

Having smaller goals helps keep up your morale because there is nothing like achieving that first milestone. That is when you know you are on the right path, and it makes you want to get to the next milestone.

It also keeps you in a positive can-do mindset as once you have reached the next few, you are well on your way to the final goal post.

## A New Daily Routine

When you change your eating habits, it affects your daily routine, especially when intermittent fasting. You have to schedule your meals around your fasting days as well as your social calendar. If you are unsure if you will be able to resist temptation, it is best to schedule family outings, lunches, and get-togethers on non-fasting days. There are, obviously, going to be times when you cannot do this. Instead, try to be flexible regarding your scheduled fasting days instead.

### Your Daily To-Do List

You need to organize your schedule in order to start a new routine. The first thing you should do is create your daily task list. This is everything you do throughout the day and which days you do what tasks on.

While fasting should not interfere with your daily routine, it could possibly interfere with your social one. In order to benefit from intermittent fasting, you need to make it fit into your life. To choose or modify a plan to best suit your needs, you need to establish what your current routine is so you can adapt it to fit your new lifestyle.

While jotting down what all you do during the day each day, here are some questions to keep in mind:

- How does the morning start? Write down the general time you get up. Any pre-breakfast tasks?
- Do you make breakfast every morning?
- Do you have kids you need to get off to school, college, or work?
- Do you have a partner that needs to get off to work?

- If you are working, what is your morning routine to get ready?
- Do you have any work function commitments in the next one to three months?
- Do you have any social or family functions/gatherings/commitments within the next three months?
- When are grocery days?
- When are laundry days?
- What housework do you do and when?
- Do you exercise? If so, how frequently?
- What hobbies do you have?
- Do you have a club membership and are there any club engagements coming up?
- List any events you may have coming up, holidays, sports tournaments, sport commitments, and so on.

Include everything that you may think is relevant to your schedule that you know you do like clockwork. Events such as weddings, engagement parties, birthday functions, work functions all need to be jotted down. As do any social engagements, book clubs, girls' nights out, etc. They all play a crucial part in having a well-adjusted fasting schedule that works well with and for you.

## Create a New Schedule

Choose the type of fasting plan you think you may be able to start with and stick to. Before you commit to time windows for fasting and eating, assess your current schedule. You will need to adjust your schedule and maybe even modify your fasting plan to find a compromise for your schedule.

Before you start making up your schedule, it is time to take stock of you. Note the times of day you feel you have the highest energy levels. This is the time of day to do the heavy lifting, like exercises and training your mind to break old habits to make room for new ones. Use your afternoons to set up menus for the next day, make appointments, go watch the kid's sports games or meet up with friends for tea.

Do things that do not require a lot of energy, but that still keep you active and your mind working.

You should include a number of things on your schedule like:

- The time you need to wake up each morning so you can set your alarm.
- Any appointments you, your partner, or kids may have each day.
- Shopping for groceries, or any household, school, or office supplies you may need.
- Family commitments for the day or evening.

- Upcoming events you need to get yourself and your family ready for.
- New foods you would like to try each day.
- Any changes you would like to make on certain days that will ease you into your new healthy lifestyle.
- Exercise for the day.
- Set a time window for bedtimes. This may seem a bit infantile, but you need to start getting a decent sleep pattern going. If you make a concerted effort to get to bed at a regular time each night, your body will soon adapt to this routine. You will find yourself starting to feel tired by a certain point of the evening.

### *Wake Up with a Smile*

The most popular time of day for high-energy levels is when you first wake up. This is the time your body should be well-rested and restored. This is the time of day you should be the most active and enjoy your energy. Make the most of the time to go for a walk, get the major part of your tasks done before your energy levels start to get depleted.

Train yourself to wake up with the correct attitude. Wake up with the first ring of your alarm — do not hit that snooze button. Have a big stretch to get the blood flowing through your system and get up, don't be tempted to laze in your bed. Your attitude upon waking will set the tone for the entire day.

Not everyone is a morning person but resetting the alarm is resetting your brain into old habits. It is as if you are putting off waking up for the day and you need to change that to be more positive. Even if you feel a bit blah at first, take a deep breath, stretch and hop out of bed. Smile if only to yourself in the mirror as a smile is infectious and makes everyone feel better.

A refreshing shower is a good way to get yourself going in the morning and it makes you feel alive. It is a symbolic way to wash away the sleepiness from the night before and step out of the shower cleansed for the new day. Splashing cold water on your face and neck will stimulate the Vagus nerve and kick start your morning as well.

### Be Active Throughout the Day

You may not feel like it as your energy levels start to get depleted but don't slow down altogether. Don't take an afternoon nap either, that may just make you feel even more lethargic and can cause problems by disturbing your nightly sleep patterns.

If you work in an office environment, take a break every thirty minutes where you actually get up and go get a glass of water. Stand up and stretch, roll your neck, and stretch out your feet. Get your blood pumping through your veins and take some deep breaths.

If you are at home, go for a walk around the garden and check out your plants. Or go for a walk in the park, feed the ducks and take in some fresh air. Do a puzzle or play Candy Crush for fifteen minutes to get your brain stimulated as well.

As long as you are keeping your mind ticking and pushing through the feeling of lethargy that may creep up on you in the afternoons. If you can push through it, you will eventually find you will start to have a little more afternoon energy each afternoon.

Going for a swim and getting some gentle exercise even when you feel like your body just wants to collapse is a good way to get the adrenaline flowing through your system. If you must close your eyes, have a small five- to eight-minute power nap. You will be surprised how refreshed you can feel when you close your eyes and let yourself relax for shorter periods of time.

### The Evenings

It is important to make evenings the time of day when you put away all the stress and anxieties of the day. When you walk through the front door or notice the clock turn six, it is time to shut out the day. Concentrate on what you have to do in the evening, like getting supper going, change into comfortable clothes, and maybe get ready for the next day.

Once you have had your evening meal, which you should try to eat by 7:30 pm each day, plan your next day. Decide on your meals, get your clothes ready, take a shower to wash off the day then take time to relax. Watch a bit of TV or read a good book or just have a chat with your partner and kids.

Make evenings about family, you, and getting organized for tomorrow. Leave the worrying about the next day for the next day. Evenings are the time you need to learn to unwind to allow for good quality sleep. When you do not get enough sleep, it makes it difficult to successfully fast, or get through your next day.

### Give Yourself Room to Be Flexible

Having a set routine is a good thing but that does not mean you have to be completely rigid with it. Remember to give yourself a little bit of room for error. Your body needs to adjust to its new lifestyle so give yourself some time. Keep an open mind and learn how to quickly adjust and adapt to any situations that may arise.

You can have your routines and comfort zones but don't forget to be a little spontaneous too. Life is not all boring mundane routines it is also about living and during your golden years is the time to enjoy life.

Let go once in a while, listen to your body and follow its lead.

Setting up new routines is going to take getting used to. Some things may not work at first so adjust them until they do work for you and you find them easy to follow. Changing your mindset is not about creating problems or making life more difficult for you. It is about finding a new balance that works just as smoothly as the old one did. Only the new one is setting you up for a new healthier you with clean eating habits.

Deep down we all wish we could have a perfect life that ran smoothly like clockwork. But the reality is that life can be messy and no matter how perfectly we plan it, it does not always go according to plan. Keep your goals and schedules real, achievable and flexible. You cannot plan for everything, but there are certain things that you can plan for. The things that you can't, you will have to deal with as they happen. As you adjust to a healthier lifestyle, you will find the unexpected a lot easier to deal with without the foggy brain or run-down feeling.

Those things you can plan for, you don't need to set them in stone, just have a good idea of how you are going to deal with them.

## It Is All Up to You

Reading self-help books, laying out the groundwork, and setting goals is the easy part. The hard part is putting it all into practice and that is all up to you. Now that you have chosen your fasting plan, decided upon a diet, and set your new routine, it is time to take the next step.

It is time to get real and set a realistic start date. Go to bed the night before and think about sleep as your cocoon. The next morning you are going to wake up taking on the first day of your new lifestyle. The new you is about to start blossoming and become healthier, stronger, and more confident.

# Chapter 11: Reaching Your Goals

It takes a lot of hard work and staying power. Once you have reached your goal weight, dropped a dress size or two there is no greater feeling.

## You Made It!

When you have come so far, it is cause for celebration and everyone deserves to have a bit of fun, let their hair down and reward themselves. As long as you do not fall back into old habits and keep a maintenance plan that maintains your weight as well as your health.

## You Are What You Eat

When you have reached your goal weight, you will feel healthier, have more energy, and look great. You may even have a glow about you as your system is cleansed and has probably been kick-started to work at its optimum level. Be mindful of what you eat and keep up the good habits of grabbing the healthier options of your favorite foods.

## New Lifestyle, New You

A healthier lifestyle is the best change you can make. Your healthier choices and intermittent fasting lifestyle will become the new you. You may not be the same girl you once were, but now you are an incredible woman. You are stronger, more confident and a whole lot healthier.

## Enjoy Your Success

When you feel good you will look good and will be able to wear your new-found confidence with pride. And you earned it so enjoy your midlife years, they are nothing to be ashamed of but rather are to be enjoyed. You have passed all the awkward years, you are over all of your insecurities, and now you get to be you. A new, gorgeous, healthier you that glows from the inside out.

# Chapter 12: Getting Started

Starting a diet is a challenge because as soon as you register the word diet it becomes a mission. You have an instant mental block towards it and you may even start to crave things you normally do not eat on a regular basis. The most popular day for a diet to start is tomorrow. Don't get caught in that trap and eat all you can today thinking you are going to start the diet tomorrow.

Even thinking about a lifestyle change can send your subconscious into self-preservation and rebellious mode. It is easy for others to say get over yourself and do it, but a person gets set in their ways and for years they follow their daily patterns. Now all of a sudden there are big changes on the horizon and let's face it no one likes to change. Especially change that means turning your lifestyle upside down like a diet does.

## Getting Ready to Embrace Your New Lifestyle

Before you get started there are a few things you should do and may need to get ready.

### Speak to a Medical Professional

This is very important if you are on any kind of medication. If you have a pre-existing condition or are ill in any way, you should not try fasting without the guidance of a medical professional.

It is a good idea to get a medical checkup before you start a diet. Even young adults should always start a diet getting the all-clear from a doctor.

### *Choose a Fasting Plan*

If you are starting out with intermittent fasting, choose a plan that is not too limiting. For instance, the 5:2 plan with a 12-hour fasting period and a 12-hour eating window to begin with. You could try the 16-hour fasting period and 8-hour eating window if you think you will cope.

If you find the plan is too much for you, switch it for another one or modify the one you are on. Build yourself up to a longer fasting period. As long as you are moving forward and not going backward with your fasting plan.

**Set achievable goals** and make sure you give yourself some wiggle room as well as being prepared for the times you may slip.

**Make a calendar** and place it where you can see it, mark your fasting and non-fasting days as well as time windows on it.

**Keep an intermittent fasting diary**, log how you felt during fasting, any changes you have found within yourself, improvements, days you may have fallen off the fasting wagon. It is important to document the process as it demonstrates your commitment and it will inspire you.

**Be kind to yourself**, you are going to have unpleasant days and good days. It is important to remember you are doing this for you. Don't feel guilty for one guilty pleasure now and then, just ensure they become less and less frequent..

## Fasting Diet Plan

The best diet during the fasting period is to only drink unsweetened, carb-free drinks like water, tea, and coffee. But there is nothing wrong with starting out with a 500 calorie allowance during the fasting period. Most people find it easier to fast through the night into the late morning.

## Non-Fasting Day Eating Plan

Although there is no recommended diet for intermittent fasting, it is advisable to follow a healthy clean eating plan. Cut down on daily calorie intake, drink more water and choose fruit or nuts instead of sugary or processed foods. Make small changes and start switching out the unhealthy for more natural healthier products. Don't overthink the process and slowly you will rewire your brain to automatically reach for those foods.

Some good eating plans are a low-carb diet, calorie cycling plans like Weight Watchers, and becoming more aware of what you are eating. Make a point of thinking that you are what you eat, and you want to be healthy.

*Breakfast*

It has been drilled into a person since youth that breakfast is the most important meal of the day. But that does not mean you can't eat it at say 11 am; you are still eating breakfast.

It is believed that breakfast kick starts a person's metabolism to aid in the burning of calories throughout the day. There are other ways to kick start your metabolism like including a dash of cayenne pepper to your morning coffee. Cayenne pepper helps the body to burn calories for up to three hours after consuming it. First, check with your doctor before using it as it can interfere with some medical conditions and medications.

In general, it is not going to harm you to skip breakfast a few times a week during a fasting period. Our ancestors did not get up every morning to a bowl of porridge or a three-egg omelet. Your body will soon adjust to its new routine, and you will start missing your morning meal less.

## Charged with Optimism

"Whatever the mind can conceive and believe, the mind can achieve" — (Hill, 1937).

Start your new intermittent fasting lifestyle off on an optimistic note. Go into the diet fully charged and ready to go. Psych yourself up mentally and enthusiastically think of this change as going on a holiday from the old you and embrace this journey you have embarked upon.

If you believe you can do it, you will do it. Just keep pushing through the tough days, enjoy the good days, and forgive the slip-ups. Eventually, you will be having more good days than bad until you have completely turned your lifestyle around and are reaping the benefits of it.

# Conclusion

Intermittent fasting can be very challenging at first but if you can get over the few times and stick to it, it is immensely rewarding.

Don't give up if you feel that the fasting plan you have chosen is too much for you. Ask your medical advisor to help you either modify your current plan or try another one. Not everyone is suited to each plan. You may find you need to try one or two before you are comfortable.

You don't have to dive right into adjusting your eating habits as well as try intermittent fasting all at once either. Start off fasting, eating normally but cutting down and gradually make food choice changes as you become more comfortable with fasting.

The trick is to find your balance, one step at a time if you must, as long as you are working to your end goal. How long it takes to get you there is entirely up to you. Don't think you have to rush headlong into it. Set achievable realistic goals that you feel one hundred percent comfortable with, otherwise your intermittent fasting diet is not going to work.

This is a lifestyle change, not a fad diet that you try for a few days or weeks and then forget because it became mundane or too challenging. This is a diet and lifestyle you need to commit to that will not only help you lose weight but be beneficial for your health. There is nothing wrong with easing into it; it is not a race and you have to remember you are doing this for you!

Well done on your decision to make a choice to try the intermittent fasting and all the very best. You can do this — you have got this!

# References

9 Ways to Eat Clean. (2018, February 22). Retrieved from
https://www.webmd.com/diet/ss/slideshow-how-to-
eat-clean

Anapanasati. (n.d.). [PDF File] Retrieved from
http://www.buddhanet.net/pdf_file/anapanasati.pdf

Arguin, H., Dionne, I. J., Sénéchal, M., Bouchard, D. R.,
Carpentier, A. C., Ardilouze, J.-L., ... Brochu, M. (2012,
August). Short- and long-term effects of continuous
versus intermittent restrictive diet approaches on body
composition and the metabolic profile in overweight and
obese postmenopausal women: a pilot study. Retrieved
from
https://www.ncbi.nlm.nih.gov/pubmed/22735163Barna
, M. (2019, January 02). The science behind fasting
diets. Retrieved from
https://www.discovermagazine.com/health/fasting-
may-be-more-than-a-fad-diet

Barnosky, A., Hoddy, K., Unterman, T. & Varady, K. (2014,
October 01). Intermittent fasting vs daily calorie
restriction for type 2 diabetes prevention: a review of
human findings. Retrieved from
https://www.sciencedirect.com/science/article/pii/S193
152441400200X

Benefits of Intermittent Fasting for Women Over 50. (2019, September 03). Retrieved from https://primewomen.com/health/nutrition/benefits-of-intermittent-fasting-for-women-over-50/

Catterjee, S. (2016, January 01). Chapter two - Oxidative stress, inflammation, and disease. Retrieved from https://www.sciencedirect.com/science/article/pii/B9780128032695000024

Cole, W. (2017, November 09). The impact intermittent fasting can have on all your hormones. Retrieved from https://drwillcole.com/the-impact-intermittent-fasting-can-have-on-all-your-hormones/

Cronkleton, E. (2018, August 15). Taking a better breath. Retrieved from https://www.healthline.com/health/how-to-breathe

Dierks, T. (n.d.). Psychiatry research: Neuroimaging. Retrieved from https://www.journals.elsevier.com/psychiatry-research-neuroimaging/

Differential Effects of Alternate-Day Fasting Versus Daily Calorie Restriction on Insulin Resistance. (2019, September 27). Retrieved from https://www.ncbi.nlm.nih.gov/pubmed/31328895

Fasting — A History Part 1. (n.d.). Retrieved from https://thefastingmethod.com/fasting-a-history-part-i/

Fasting and Meditation: Everything You Need to Know. Retrieved from https://kenshoway.com/meditation/fasting-meditation-everything-you-need-to-know

Gunnars, K. (2018, July 25). Intermittent fasting 101 — The ultimate beginner's guide. Retrieved from https://www.healthline.com/nutrition/intermittent-fasting-guide

Hill, N. (1937). *Think and grow rich* (1937th ed.). Wise, Virginia: Napoleon Hill Foundation.

Hormones as you age. (n.d.). Retrieved from https://www.rush.edu/health-wellness/discover-health/hormones-you-age

LaBier, D. (2015, February 10). How meditation changes the structure of your brain. Retrieved from https://www.psychologytoday.com/us/blog/the-new-resilience/201502/how-meditation-changes-the-structure-your-brain

Holzel, B. K., CArmody, J., Vangel, M., Congleton, C., Yerramsetti, S. M., Gard, T., Lazar, S. W. (2011 January 30). Mindfulness practice leads to increases in regional brain gray matter density. *Psychiatry Research: Neuroimaging*. Vol 191 (1) p36-43. Retrieved from https://www.sciencedirect.com/science/article/abs/pii/S092549271000288X

Papconstantinou, J. (2019, November 04). The role of signaling pathways of inflammation and oxidative stress in the development of senescence and aging phenotypes in

cardiovascular disease. Retrieved from
https://www.mdpi.com/2073-4409/8/11/1383

Rupasinghe, V. (2016, September 22). *Oxidative medicine and cellular longevity* [PDF File]. Retrieved from
https://www.hindawi.com/journals/omcl/2016/743279
7/

Shah, A. (n.d.). Intermittent Fasting Can Heal Your Gut & Calm Inflammation. Here's Exactly How To Do It. Retrieved from https://www.mindbodygreen.com/0-28912/intermittent-fasting-can-heal-your-gut-calm-inflammation-heres-exactly-how-to-it.html

The Health Benefits of Tai Chi. (2019, August 20). Retrieved from https://www.health.harvard.edu/staying-healthy/the-health-benefits-of-tai-chi

Valter, D. & Mattson, P. (2014, February 4). Fasting: Molecular Mechanisms and Clinical Applications. Retrieved from https://www.ncbi.nlm.nih.gov/pmc/articles/PMC39461 60/

When Sciences Meets Mindfulness. (n.d.). Retrieved from https://news.harvard.edu/gazette/story/2018/04/harva rd-researchers-study-how-mindfulness-may-change-the-brain-in-depressed-patients/

www.ingramcontent.com/pod-product-compliance
Lightning Source LLC
Chambersburg PA
CBHW050727030426

42336CB00012B/1448